THE 30-DAY CAST-AWAY PROGRAM

Julia Caranci

Certified Personal Trainer

SELF-PUBLISHED IN 2018

Contents

About the Author

Julia Caranci grew up in a working class family living in a small town where opportunities were few and far between. Her family was not rich by any stretch and she was bullied at school like many other children, whether because they are too big or too little or even because their mom makes their clothes. She suffered from severe anxiety as a result, which went undiagnosed for many years. When Julia was in her early 20s, she discovered physical exercise in the form of running, weight lifting, yoga and hiking, as a means to both keep herself in shape and to combat anxiety. After several careers, including a 10-year stint as a print journalist, Julia finally achieved her goal of becoming a Personal Trainer at the age of 45. She combined her love of exercise with her love of writing and created this book to help others achieve their fitness goals. While exercise doesn't solve all life's problems, Julia strongly believes that the benefits of physical activity, combined with a good mental attitude, can help combat many of life's struggles. Julia lives on Vancouver Island with her husband and cheerleader, David, and her beautiful black cats: Magic and Smudge.

Chapter 1

A Story about Mary and the 130 lbs

I worked with a very lovely woman named Mary at an extremely busy, stressful newspaper office for seven years. When I first met Mary, she weighed more than 300 lbs and was unhappy with her life. However, she had recently made a very strong commitment to lose the weight — for once and for all — at the age of 49. She joined a gym, changed her diet and began fighting hard to get her body back.

Mary told me frankly that she had gained and lost 100 or more pounds several different times in her life, only to gain it back each time, and then some. To me, this was incredible! How can someone put themselves through such huge physical and emotional changes over and over again? Yet, it happens to be true that 97 per cent of us who lose weight gain it all back within about three years. Clearly, there's a message here. The message is that many of us know what we need to do to get fit, and may even have done what we need to do to get fit … but we just can't seem to maintain that strong, self-confident and courageous demeanour.

Mary, being a woman with not only a boatload of bravery but also a wonderful sense of humour, said her goal was, "To be skinny for more than five minutes THIS TIME."

She was fresh out of a separation from her husband and wanted badly to succeed.

Well, Mary continued going to the gym every day and monitoring her diet — and those of us who worked with her watched as, day by day and week by week, she lost weight while toning her body. It was very inspiring to many of us to see someone make real and significant changes to their life and to their body. As many of you likely already know, it's incredibly difficult to make real and significant changes to your life for reasons that I will go into later on in this book.

In about a year she had achieved an incredible feat: she lost 140 pounds of fat and stood in front of us, the slimmest she had ever been in her adult life! Dressed in slim-fitting jeans and a fitted T-shirt, Mary looked like a new woman. People who knew her and hadn't seen her in a while were just floored when they walked into the office. Compliments came her way many times a day, and she glowed in her achievement. Her ex would eat his heart out!

That was in January of 2009. Our newspaper did a very nice piece on her weight loss, and she really inspired others, helping many who were in the same situation she was in just a few months before. She was on top of the world, and she deserved to be. Mary had really made a massive shift in her life. She felt amazing about herself and firmly believed that this was her forever body.

We were all very proud of Mary and believed that her transformation was incredible. We talked about it in the halls at the office. We praised Mary whenever we saw her in a new outfit. She joked that she had finally thrown away her "fat pants" forever — put them all in a garbage bag and drove them to the dump herself. She HAD to buy an entirely new wardrobe, being that she could fit her whole body into one leg of her old pants!

Fast forward 16 months later …. Mary had put back on virtually every pound she lost. It happened in front of our eyes; just like the weight loss. At first, it seemed like she might be backsliding a bit, but surely (we thought) she would jump back on the wagon again in short order!

Then a few weeks later, I noticed her belly protruding out from under her shirts again; watched her self-consciously tugging the shirt back down over and over throughout the day. She stopped talking about her life, her weight and her progress. She wouldn't look you in the eye. We all felt a strange sense of embarrassment whenever we saw her, and the topic of weight and weight loss became taboo subjects around her. Just a few months before that was about all she wanted to talk about.

So, what happened to Mary?

Of course, we never said anything to her face. How could we? How could we broach this difficult topic with a woman who, just a few months before, was literally our fitness hero and weight loss guru?

One day Mary and I were alone in the lunch room and she began to talk to me about what happened. It started with her grabbing a 50 lb water container and doing a few squats with it — very impressive as the container was awkward and weighed more than 50 lbs.

"You certainly are very strong, Mary," I said to her.

She then told me that yes, she was, but that she had completely fallen off the wagon and felt like she had lost everything. Pretending I wasn't fully aware of this already, I asked her how that had happened?

Mary told me frankly that, after losing the weight and finally reaching her goal, she became depressed and was completely plagued by thoughts of self-doubt, fear and shame. She thought her husband would beg her to come back when he saw that she was fit and trim, but he didn't. This sent her into a mental spiral. She started to doubt herself and the fear — which had always permeated her subconscious mind — took away everything that she had achieved. In short, she stopped believing in herself, which was incredible considering that she stopped believing AFTER she had achieved all her goals.

With tears in her eyes, she said that the moment she was rejected again by her ex, she completely lost all faith in herself, and turned to food to comfort her and hide from the truth. This in turn propelled her straight back to comfort eating like she had done all her life, and she gained back all the weight that she had lost — a year's worth of extremely hard work — in just a couple of months. I was in equal parts amazed that Mary had shared her story with me, and confounded by what had happened.

It was a stunning revelation to me to hear it put so succinctly by someone who had personally experienced this yo-yo weight loss and weight gain phenomenon. Mary basically confessed that her belief in her own success was so fragile, that the moment this success wasn't mirrored back to her by her husband wanting her back, she proceeded to turn back into the fat woman she believed herself to be. The woman that was hurt and abandoned.

I tell you this story not to put a spotlight on anyone's failure (and in fact she didn't fail, she actually succeeded), but to make you understand the life lesson behind this story: If your belief in yourself isn't strong enough to weather difficult times; if you even for a moment stop believing that you deserve to be happy, fit and well; then you can easily crash back into the abyss.

What Mary needed and failed to arm herself with was that store of unshakable internal belief in herself that can only be achieved by controlling both the conscious and subconscious mind, and having both those forces constantly on guard for your own best interests. Clearly, the problem was not that Mary couldn't lose the weight.

In fact, she DID lose it, and more than one or two or even three times!

No, Mary's failure was in not having the mental strength and support to back her up and keep her on the right path for life.

Does any of this story sound like you? Have you lost, then gained weight back again more than one time? Is it scary for you to make changes to your life, even though you know that they will benefit you in the end and may even save your life? Do you get on the fitness bandwagon with the best of intentions, only to fall back into your old ways within just a couple of weeks?

Look, I understand what it's like to have to fight for your life. I know misery and unhappiness. But I also know that we can change, and change for good. Give me 30 days, and you will be well on your way to becoming an entirely new person with an unshakable set of core beliefs in yourself and in your ability to succeed no matter WHAT life throws at your.

I know what I'm talking about. I have made fitness a personal priority in my life for more than 25 years. I run, lift weights, hike, walk, practice yoga, create workout videos and constantly strive to learn more about fitness every day.

I am a Certified Personal Trainer, Ergo Assessor, Industrial First Aid Attendant, Writer and have taught myself how to grow to master my subconscious mind through meditation, study and visualization. It's much harder than you might think, but once you are in control of both your minds AND your body, you will be unstoppable.

Sound good? OK, read on ...

Chapter 2

It's all in your Mind - Really!

What if you could snap your fingers and suddenly be the fit, healthy, active person you really think you should be? Would you snap your fingers right now?

Of course, almost all of you reading this would answer "Yes, I'm not stupid, of course I would!"

But the first thing that overweight and/or unhealthy people need to consider is that just like someone who suffers from a condition like depression or anxiety (I know anxiety very well because I suffer from it), or someone who is a hoarder or stays in a damaging relationship, that there are emotional benefits and addictive feelings that go along with our current condition that make it difficult to change.

The result of these feelings is that when we try to make changes, we are often paralyzed by fear. Fear is how our subconscious mind alerts us that something is out of the ordinary. And because this part of your brain is afraid of change, it creates such a strong fear impulse in you that you often just stop before you achieve anything at all.

Your subconscious is the part of your brain that acts in large part without you even knowing. It drives the car while you think about work or a recent argument; it breaths and chews and walks and reacts for you without you consciously deciding to — in fact most experts now agree that 97 per cent of our habits and behaviours are controlled by our subconscious mind. The good part about this is that we don't have to think about how to drive a car or breath or duck — the bad part is that this part of your brain has recorded both all the good and ALL the bad things that have ever happened to you. It has developed opinions for you on things that you may not consciously agree with. However, when you try to change, your subconscious creates such uncomfortable physical and mental conditions (especially at first) that you often just give up — not even really knowing why. Except … now you do.

We may think and say that outside reasons are stopping us from getting out of that bad relationship or losing those 50 pounds, but in reality, we cannot separate ourselves from our problems. Our lives are an utterly perfect reflection of every choice we have made in our lives from as far back as we can remember to right now; this very moment. To try to blame something or someone else for our current condition is not only incorrect, but that kind of reasoning will keep us stuck in our ruts forever.

You are by now beginning to grasp that the problem here is not so much physical, but mental. If you understand this, than you are already getting something HUGE from reading this. There are blockages — some call them limiting beliefs, others call them thinking errors — that are stopping you from making changes to your life because there is a powerful drive in your mind to keep the steady routine you are in. It's funny because if you begin to delve into the human mind and how people become truly successful and achieve miraculous things — it's mainly those who do something completely different, or who take a tremendous risk, or really put themselves out there, at risk for failure. The funny part about this is that our brains are constantly trying to tell us NOT to take these kind of risks and just to keep doing the same thing over and over and over again. But if you look at any person who has ultimately achieved something immense with their lives, they undoubtedly describe a long series of failures that ultimately led to success. You cannot succeed unless you are willing and open to failing first.

Your subconscious mind is behind this, because it is not ok with change — it likes routine because it feels like you are being protected from anything dangerous when things stay nice and predictable. Again, let's talk about driving your car. Your subconscious mind makes a lot of your decisions while you are driving, and the rest of you follows along. You certainly wouldn't want to do anything unpredictable or unexpected while you were driving, because that actually could put your life and safety in danger. The problem is that your subconscious acts like this no matter what part of your life is at stake. While it may be very helpful when you are driving down the highway at 80 miles an hour, it's not very helpful when you are in a rut that includes watching tv on the couch every night and never trying any new activities.

And as most motivational speakers will attest to, using mindless entertainment as a hobby really doesn't benefit your life at all.

I'm not making this up, it is a proven psychological fact. When you start a new routine, or try to break a habit that is deeply engrained inside your mind, all sorts of alarms, bells and whistles go off in your subconscious mind, and they manifest themselves into feelings that may include: fear, panic, discomfort, anxiety, depression, etc. It's very very difficult to fight off these strong feelings and push through. That's the bad news. The good news is that you CAN push through them, provided you use some very simple mental techniques — techniques that can and will allow you to change your life for the better, permanently!

And I am in no way trying to depress you or say you can't work your way out of these circumstances. You absolutely can. People do remarkable things and rise up from seemingly hopeless circumstances to become famous and beloved. These kinds of people are literally living proof that you can rise well beyond your current condition and achieve anything that you desire — if you are willing to go for it with every fibre of your being and to never, ever give up on your dreams. Is having everything that you want worth fighting through some discomfort? Is it worthwhile to know that fear of change is completely normal but that you can overcome it? The answer to both questions is YES!

Consider Booker T. Washington, an African American man who was born into a family of slaves and subjected to very poor and meagre beginnings in life. He was literally put to work in a salt mine while still a very young boy, and during the days while he worked in the hot, dusty mine, he watched out the window at other little children walking back and forth from school, the one place he desperately wanted to go. He initially could not read or write, and his step-father tried to make him work instead of going to school so that the family could have the additional income. How easy would it be for someone like him to believe he had a bright future ahead of him as a famous author and civil rights advocate? He could have simply sunk into a deep depression and carried on living out his days working in a salt mine, as many many others born into similar conditions did. But that did not happen. In his amazing book chronicling his childhood, he talks about how he believed, with every fibre of his being, that he would somehow go to school and learn to read and write, although there was nothing in his present circumstances that even hinted that this was even a possibility. Anyone who had heard him say this as a young black boy working in a salt mine with absolutely no education to speak of would have thought it near impossible.

But Booker T. Washington did educate himself. In fact, he became a writer, intellectual and civil rights activist in his own lifetime, along with helping countless other poor men and women in similar circumstances also become educated and better themselves. Throughout his writings, Booker simply asserts that his motivation was that he believed deeply in his own ability to succeed in getting an education, and he simply would not allow the idea of failure to enter into his consciousness. Instead of believing that his current existence was all he could hope for, he created a new vision of what he wanted his life to be, and set about making that a reality one small step at a time. This is what can happen to someone who is able to overcome their own negative thought patterns and their subconscious belief system. If Booker could do what he did with his life, then you CAN lose 25, 50, 100 or more pounds of fat, if you first change how you feel about yourself, then begin doing something about it. If you believe in yourself, it doesn't matter what your body looks like now, or how fit you are currently, all that will matter is that you take that one small step at a time to make the changes that will bring you the body that you want and deserve to have.

Step One: Finding out the fears that are holding you back — which usually can be traced back to one or more limiting beliefs that you may have about yourself. There are a number of limiting beliefs, but some of the main ones that are engrained into our subconscious minds as children are: I am not worthy; I can't do (fill in the blank); If I try to really be me I will be rejected; nothing ever works out for me; I am stupid.

The only way to really pinpoint which limiting beliefs are holding you back from achieving your fitness goals is to really pay attention to your thoughts and your reactions to people and situations. My therapist told me, during one of our first sessions together, that you can measure being upset about something on a scale of one to 10 - one being floating down a placid river on a beautiful summer day and 10 being in a full-blown rage screaming your face off at someone who has just dealt you a horrible emotional blow. She said that well adjusted people will RARELY go beyond a 3 out of 10 on that scale.

I was pretty floored by that to be honest. Because I had spent much of my adult life getting well above a three on a daily basis over things that seemed important at the time, but really just weren't. In other words, I began to understand that I did not truly have control over my thoughts and feelings — and having this kind of control is really the only way you can begin to control your life, your body and how you treat it. The things that were constantly upsetting me came from a deep abyss inside myself. While there are a small number of people in the world who are completely well adjusted and had a perfect childhood, the vast majority of us have internal scars that manifest themselves in how we treat ourselves and other people in our lives.

I can relate strongly to feeling bad about yourself and having limiting beliefs about yourself. I grew up in a home with an extremely fearful and overprotective mother, and a verbally, emotionally and physically abusive father. I never knew from one day to the next what my dad might do to me, or to my mother or siblings. That kind of upbringing is marked by instability. The result? I grew up and became an extremely anxious woman who bounced from relationship to relationship and job to job, never truly realizing why I was doing the things I was doing. I lost my temper a lot, burned bridges with family, friends, bosses and co-workers, and blamed other people for the resulting problems in my life. It was only in my forties that I begin to get some real therapy, and meditate and begin to consider that I could fundamentally change myself, starting from the depths of my subconscious beliefs about myself. And the first step was understanding that no one else but me is responsible for my life and for making myself successful and happy. Whatever happened to me as a child made its mark, to be sure, however where I would take the rest of my life was entirely up to me.

It's like that famous question therapists ask: what would you do if you didn't have your story — who would you be?

By "story" they mean the past until now — the collection of experiences, particularly growing up, that help to shape and form us into the adults we become, upon which are heaped plenty of other good — and no so good — experiences. This whole heap of stuff is what gets piled on top of the real person underneath it all — and sometimes the real and authentic you is smothered. The problem with that we lose this tiny little real part of us at the bottom of the pile — this diamond. A perfect, holy and true part of us that we really should be in touch with and reflecting all the time. So the point of the question is that if you could wake up tomorrow and you didn't have any of your baggage to carry around — if none of the bad things that happened to you were imprinted on you any longer, who would — who could — you suddenly be? Think about you without your hangups, habits, fears, routines, limits and pre-existing beliefs about what you can do with your own life and how far you might go?

This opens up a world of opportunities for us as a powerful tool for thinking about and making change. I am an English Major who become a newspaper journalist and then a personal trainer, it all sounds good on paper, but I have had many roadblocks along the way and faced many challenges. Often these challenges were things I did to sabotage myself.

When I was 43 years old I bought a house that turned from my dream home into a complete nightmare. During a heavy rainstorm the bottom floor of my home flooded and I spent an entire night bailing water my myself, desperate to save the house that I had purchased just five weeks before. For the first few days and weeks after I met with insurance adjusters, restoration specialists, floor layers, etc etc, trying to put the broken pieces of the puzzle back together. I almost walked away from my home entirely. Fortunately my caring neighbour and friend talked me out of that.

The thing was that even after the renovations got done, I still felt the trauma of the night of the flooding. Something had gotten stuck in my brain and just wouldn't leave me in peace.

- I began seeing a very good therapist who helped change my life, and has inspired me to make REAL changes, to have REAL successes and in turn, to make me want to share those lessons with anyone who decides they are sick and tired of making the same mistakes over and over again. As it turned out, it was not what had happened to me that was the real problem (because floors and walls can be fixed), It was how my subconscious mind was behaving that was the problem

This is a book about changing your body by changing your mind, first and foremost. It's a book about fitness and ways to help you become fit by training first your mind and then yourself with useful tools and tips I will provide in upcoming chapters.

I will share with you some very useful tools therapists use to help you improve your life by helping you develop tricks and tips to bring your subconscious around to being ON YOUR SIDE. I am not a therapist. I am only going to share common sense tools that worked for me, and may also help you along your goal to physical and mental fitness, as we can't really have one without the other and consider ourselves happy. It's no fun to have a fat covered body over a beautiful personality, but a beautiful body over an unhappy inside also brings us no closer to real joy — no closer to digging out the real us under all that goop.

Over the following chapters in this book, I am going to give you short lessons on the things I have learned from experience that work to help you get fitter in mind and body, then encourage you to take those snippets, do your own research and become your own trainer, your own life coach.

Think of this book as a series of short life lessons that I have learned — try them on — not all of the ideas and practices will work for you, but they are all based on facts and I would really like to help people become who they really — the reason why I am going to provide lessons on how to train your body interposed with how to train your mind, is because by doing both, you will give yourself the best chance at success. Also, I would have really, really loved it if someone had taken me on this journey 20 or even 10 years ago — not that I am not grateful to have it now — but only to say you are never too young (nor too old) to unlearn the bad, re-learn the good and get on the road to being far happier with both your body.... And your mind.

Chapter 3
Start by Stopping
(How you Talk to Yourself)

I work with many women in an office setting now — and I am completely blown away at the violent and hateful way some women talk about themselves — out loud — to not just themselves, but to other people. It shocks me because these women have no idea how hard they are being on themselves, and how damaging talking to yourself badly is, how it can completely sabotage your efforts to start working on becoming fit. Here are some real examples of things women I know and respect, who maybe have a bit of weight to lose but are not, by any means, obese, talk about themselves to others:

"I can't wear tights, I'm so fat that I can't stand the way my ass looks in them."

"I'm not pretty like you girls, I could never look sexy."

"I am so fat, I can't stand it."

"I could never be skinny like you."

Really, if I could give anyone a starting off tip to beginning a fitness program and thinking about and planning to make real change, it would be this: Stop saying bad things about yourself — firstly, out loud, and secondly, every time you catch yourself thinking bad things about yourself, just stop. Say it out loud - Stop,

Julia. Stop thinking about that — let's think about this instead - I'm going for a walk after work, I'm going to the gym tomorrow morning, I'm eating a very good meal tonight, I used to be more fit so I can become that way again.

At the same time as you are cleaning out your cupboards of junk food, researching a gym you might like to join, announcing your intention to get fit to friends and family and asking them for support, you need to be really paying attention to how you speak to yourself. Honestly, the best thing you can do is ask your family and friends to stop you — dead in your tracks — whenever they hear you talking trash about yourself. Look: no one else in life is here to make your life better except you. So if you aren't going to be your own greatest cheerleader, then no one is! Talk

To yourself like you would talk to someone you really cared about — talk to yourself like you would talk to a best friend. Honestly, before you can really successfully change your life, you need to look in the mirror and start helping out that beautiful soul staring back at you.

The next best thing you can do to Cast-Away that inner critic who is holding you down is to begin researching some positive meditations and self-hypnosis videos from U-Tube and begin downloading and listening to ones that strike a cord in you.

Look, whether you realize it or not, your subconscious mind is actually running the show. It's the larger part of your brain power hidden behind your conscious mind that is actually making decisions for you because it has engrained in your brain set ideas about what you like to do, what you like to eat, what routines you stick to and what it thinks is good for you.

However …. The problem with our subconscious mind running the show for us is that it's rubric's cube of ideas about who it thinks you are were formed during the very early years of your life, when you had little control over the people who raised you, educated you and told you how the world was. And if like so many of us, those ideas were somehow flawed, then you, like me, are stuck inside thinking patterns that you may not ever question or change, unless you are reading this book!

Whether you realize it or not, your brain runs on a huge storehouse of information — like a big filing cabinet — of things you have seen, heard, read or learned in the past — right from infancy to present day. All this information is stored in the subconscious mind. A lot of the things you believe about the world and about yourself are stored inside this filing cabinet. This is an excellent way to look at yourself — now consider the fact that some of the information in this filing cabinet is incredibly factual and useful — it's stuff you learned in school or lessons taught to you by mentors — then there's stuff that was programmed into your mind that really has no business being there — think of it as the useless paper inside a filing cabinet that really needs to be shredded — because it is useless and taking up room. This may include negative things you believe about yourself because of something someone unkind said to you, or maybe a parent or teacher not meaning to hurt your feelings said something to you — or maybe it's information you heard on the radio or saw on television. Our brains are computers that record information whether or not we consciously remember it or not. Some of the information is incredibly useful and other stuff is just garbage. We can't Shred stuff that is in our minds. But what we can do is replace the negative messages with positive ones, because both negative and positive cannot exist in our minds at the same time.

Stay with me, you want some magic tips that will make you thin and that's why you spent good money on this book. But you will never spend more than five minutes as a "skinny" person until you begin to believe that you deserve to be healthy and happy forever.

Begin by understanding that the start of any new routine will scare you. Change starts off terrorizing us, then feels like way to much work, and then eventually it becomes a new habit that doesn't cause us bad feelings at all.

Change is extremely frightening because our subconscious mind literally freaks out when you start expanding the parameters of what it thinks are your normal behaviours. I'm not a psychiatrist so I can't explain all the complex reasons why the brain tries to keep us stuck, but I do know that it does. And that's why, if you don't stick to a routine until it starts to feel normal, there is a great likelihood that you will give up on yourself simply because of mental discomfort. Think about starting a new job — it's the same type of discomfort. It lasts a few weeks to a few months and after that the vast majority of us get into what we call a "comfort zone" at work, and forget all about how hard it was those first few weeks. Remember your first day at the job you are in now? Remember how scared you were? How you thought you would never learn it all? Maybe you even felt like quitting. Fast forward to six months later and you are doing most things subconsciously and don't even really have to think about them anymore. Kind of amazing to think about.

The thing about a job is that we are usually highly motivated to stay committed through this difficult phase because we need the reward that the job pays us: money. In many cases we need it badly enough to keep going even through a lot of mental and in some cases emotional discomfort. Or maybe we went to school for a lot of years to get this job. Whatever the reason, high motivation forces us to carry on through the barriers and most of us end up comfortable where we once felt frightened and ill at ease. The scary new people we met are our friends. The lunch room a place to kick back in on breaks, not to be afraid to go in because you don't know anyone. EVERYTHING changes if you stay with the new routine.

Take this lesson very seriously into other parts of your life, particularly at the start of a new work out routine. You are going to feel uncomfortable at first — there is nothing wrong with you! You are going to want to quit and you are going to feel a very strong urge to give up. The best thing you can do for yourself, if you take no other advice in this book, is to push through those feelings of discomfort until you feel that your new lifestyle is routine and fits into your regular life. In real terms, this usually only takes three weeks to a month. This is exactly why 95% of the people who join the gym Jan. 1 are gone by Feb 1 - they are not able to make it through those first few weeks of, not even so much physical, but emotional and mental discomfort. Try to remember that its like starting a new job.

Visualization Exercise: re-framing your ideas about yourself

When I was trying to change careers and move from a dreary office job to a successful personal trainer and writer, I had a lot of difficulty making the shift. I had limiting beliefs that were holding me back. Every time I tried to make a change, I felt almost paralyzed with fear, and sometimes I made myself fail so that I wouldn't have to face quitting a job I hated to do something different.

Sounds strange, but no stranger than a person who knows what they need to do to become fitter and lose extra weight, but continue to sabotage themselves just when they are starting to make progress. But if you work on changing your mind at the same time as changing your body, I promise you that if you stick with it, you will make changes that you have never been able to make before and more than that: you will stick with it!

Try this simple visualization exercise every day for 30 days while you try begin to make changes: Take 15 minutes at the beginning of each day and sit in a quiet and peaceful space. Try to do this before you get up and drink coffee, shower, etc, because once your mind starts being stimulated by the outside world, it's much more difficult to quiet your mind. Start by closing your eyes. Breathe in and out slowly at least 10 times and try to focus on nothing but the sound and feeling of the breath going in and out of your body. After about a minute, you will begin to feel calm, focussed and intent. Think of yourself as a being that is connected to every other person, animal and life-form on the planet and feel connected to the billions of lives that exist all around you.

Next, pretend you are watching a movie about your life, and that a new scene is starting. That scene is today. In that scene you watch yourself go to the gym then out for a walk. While you are working out in the gym you see how happy you are to be finally making progress.

Imagine what your new body looks like, and the outfit you are wearing. Now go into your own body and really feel how good that feels. Watch yourself moving from machine to machine at the gym, and see yourself being really comfortable in this environment. People are coming in and they know you and say hi. You have gym friends because you're a regular now, and that feels good.

Now you are watching yourself on a brisk walk and you are smiling, maybe a friend is walking with you and you are walking and talking together. Really feel how good it feels to be physical, to be outside in the fresh air, to feel those calories burning off.

Now change the scene and picture yourself in six months from today. You walk into the gym and you are looking much more fit, confident and slender. Really feel the pride inside you that you have made this kind of progress. Really understand inside yourself that the only thing you had to do to make this happen was to repeat what you did the first day over and over again. Feel what it feels like to have this strong and slender body. Know that this is happening to you, not in the future, but right now. Feel the immense gratitude that you have overcome your battle to be fit and say to yourself — out loud — "I am so grateful that I have achieved my fitness goals and that I am 100 per cent committed to my body today and every day. I make it so and let it go."

There are a number of sites on Tube that offer help with retraining your subconscious mind - One I particularly find helpful is Your Youinverse. It offers a number of exercises you can do to help re-train your subconscious mind to be on your side.

A couple of things that are really helpful in starting out on this journey are: it's difficult to change your subconscious mind using your conscious mind — it's like a computer trying to fix a problem with its own programming — damn near impossible. However, there are a number of little tricks that can assist you in casting away the old thoughts you have about yourself that are holding you back from becoming the fit person you want and deserve to be! Remember: it's not, in most cases, clearly a physical issue; there are mental blocks or beliefs that are holding you back.

Back to these tricks: there are certain times when your subconscious mind is more amenable to change. One of these times in during meditation, which is really quiet time when you focus on nothing except your own breath and how it feels to be inside your body observing your thoughts.

The next easiest time to change how you think is during the minutes between sleeping and waking, either when you first wake up in the morning and have not yet been bombarded with stimulation, and the time right before you fall asleep at night. These are optimum times to listen to 'I am' messages, guided meditations or any inspiring messages. Once you begin to change your subconscious mind's beliefs and steer them more towards what you want to be instead of the programming you were helpless against as a child, you will begin to truly believe in yourself and face the real reasons why you aren't as fit as you want to be.

Chapter 4
Excuses: Tall Tales we Tell Ourselves!

I have been working out for 25 years and working in offices for almost the same amount of time. And if there is one thing that I have learned over that time — it's that excuses are the little lies we tell ourselves instead of taking action. The problem is — those little lies add up day after day after day and before you know it — those little lies have defined you and made you into something you didn't want to be — overweight, depressed, anxious, unhappy. These lies stem from negative beliefs we have about ourselves, that are guiding towards derailing our own attempts at becoming fit.

Crystal was a friend of mine who clearly had a weight problem, and was in fairly deep denial about it. She was famous for stopping and starting work out programs — all gung ho for about a week, then she would just stop talking about them and fall right off the wagon. She always had excuses for each time she gave up on working out after just a few days.

Sometimes she stopped working out because she got a cold or felt like she might be coming down with a cold. Sometimes it was that her knee was bothering her (probably related to being overweight) or she had a headache, or she didn't want to spend money on a gym or trainer (yet spent a fortune on hair, make-up and shoes).

I am going to let you in on a secret that all fit people and most successful people in general know to be a fact: Those of us who stick with something — in this case let's say a fitness program — don't make excuses or wait for motivation. Ever. I work out when I am tired, I work out when I have a headache, I work out when I am fighting a cold, I work out on holidays, I work out in the morning if I can't work out in the evening and I work out in the evening if I can't work out in the morning. Do you see what I mean? Waiting for motivation to hit you in the head is like waiting for a genie to pop out of a magic lantern and grant you three wishes…. Ain't gonna happen. You have to be the genie.

From my experience and observations and discussions with people over the years, I have come to understand that the world really is separated into

1. excuse makers and

2. doers.

The excuse makers — fitness ones — think that there is something different or special about non-excuse makers — or they think we always find it easy to work out — that we don't get tired and cranky, that we don't even have access to those excuse lists. WE DO - but we chose to override them — one day at a time — knowing that after a certain number of weeks or months of doing so, those excuses will seem weaker and weaker and pretty soon we won't pay them any mind. The best advice I can give to excuse makers is to recognize that that they come straight from your store of self-sabotaging thoughts, and that when you truly believe in yourself, you will not sacrifice a single work-out due to an excuse (not including a real reason such as having the flu or suffering from an injury). And you will begin to see what happens when excuses stop running your life. Excuses are not usually real, they are conjured by a part of your mind, determined to derail you — they are an easy way out that also alleviates guilt at the same time. But in the end, they can only hurt you. When you leave behind your excuses, you will come to realize that you are truly beginning to change.

When people talk about their weight problem, you can sense the disconnect because they talk about it like it's a problem that is separate from their own life: — "Here's me and my life and… over there … there's my weight problem — it's not really part of me. It is because of my job, my unsupportive husband, the baby I had five years ago," and, and, AND???

Honestly, if you want to get 75 per cent of the way towards achieving your goals in weight loss and in life you need to understand and believe just one thing: My weight problem is about me and no one else. I made myself this weight and no one helped me. And in reality, I am the only person who can change it. Period. If you can accept this, Bravo! You are on your way to making permanent change.

Our lives are a perfect reflection of us in every single way.

Each pound of extra weight you put on came from a thought that turned into an action (I want to eat this or that) or a thought that turned into an inaction (I don't feel like working out today because I have a headache). It seems like one choice here and one choice there … no big deal, but simply put, all those thoughts that become actions and inactions DID add up. They all added up and have made you what you are — every pound you gained you did yourself, so please don't blame anyone or anything else. It really won't help you at all in the long run, and the fact is that as long as you blame others for your problems (wrong thinking), you will feel comfortable not doing anything to change.

Remember that to be a fit person, you really need to think fit thoughts and to act on those fit thoughts each an every day. You need to see yourself as the person you want to be, at the weight you want to be at, and simply act like that person would act. Would the fit you make good food choices? Yes! Then do that every day, starting today. Would the fit you exercise every day? Yes! Then do that every day starting from today as well. Do you see where I am going with this? You got yourself overweight one day and one thought at a time, so get yourself fit one thought and one day at a time.

It's really about attacking negative beliefs about yourself, because no one else can do it for you. If you are an excuse maker, you are likely suffering from negative beliefs about yourself that are holding you back. I speak from personal experience. While I always worked out — mainly to help cope with my extreme anxiety and panic attacks - I did make many many mistakes. I was in many destructive relationships with men because I did not feel that I was worth loving (from my father) and was full of fears around trusting other people (from my mother). God love our parents who did the best they could, but they unintentionally imbedded core beliefs into our subconscious minds that affect how we feel about ourselves unless or until we do something about it.

 Another helpful method for me was Cognitive Behavioural Therapy, which helped me identify and dispute many of the negative feelings I had about myself. The same holds true for those of you who are hiding beneath a layer of body fat — there are limiting beliefs you have about yourself that can and will sabotage you. Work with a therapist if you can, or begin to do some research on CBT - it's something you can do on your own with books or for free simply by doing courses over the internet. Often a key exercise is realizing you may believe some of these things about yourself and not even know it.

I can't do anything right

I have no time for xxx

If only I had xxx, then xxx wouldn't have happened

I will never reach my goals

I just can't do xxxx

If you can take the courageous step of identifying which of these or other negative statements you believe about yourself, then you can begin to use affirmations, meditations, and other exercises to help turn those beliefs into positive statements. As a wise monk said: when a glass of water has been sullied by salt, the cure is not to throw out the glass of water, but to add fresh water to it until the salt is so diluted that it no longer affects the taste. In other words, you can only cure negative thoughts by replacing them with positive ones until the negative ones are drowned out.

Practice speaking positively about yourself every day, meditate every day, get yourself a good therapist if you can afford one, talk to yourself in the same way you would talk to a very good friend who you really cared about — always. Stop yourself whenever you are being abusive to yourself — turn it around and actually try to be gentle with yourself, and tell yourself that you will get there — because I believe that you will!

Chapter 5

When you Begin to Believe, then Do…

Let's get down to some basic tips that are practical for anyone who feels they are ready to care about themselves enough to start getting fit.

So many times I see training going on inside gyms and I fear they are destined to fail. I am no expert, but I know that spending 40 minutes of your hour with a trainer and talking more than working out is not going to help you feel better about yourself. I also know that a woman with 70 lbs to lose is not going to see noticeable results from 30 minutes of weight training three times a week throwing around 5 lb dumbbells. Personal trainers are taught how to create programs, but often people slip into a rut of high rep, low weight gym routines that deny the obvious: the best recipe to get someone on board with fitness is cardiovascular exercise. Slow to medium intensity cardiovascular exercise burns fat. Period.

So why are so many people flinging tiny weights around and paying good money to do so when they really need to get outside and do something? Mainly because they want to put the responsibility of them getting fit onto someone else. This also gives you someone else to blame when you quit. Several women I know have told me that they had to give up working out because personal trainers were just too expensive. But this really isn't the reason.

These same women buy shoes and clothes and get their hair done to try to feel good about themselves. Fact is that when you don't see fast progress, you make an excuse to fire your trainer. Really it's about getting the right kind of training, which in our modern age can be free or almost free, provided you have access to UTUBE.

In reality, it doesn't cost much money to start a cardio hobby like walking, running, swimming, biking, roller blading, cross country skiing ... and the list goes on. A warm jacket and some runners can start you off nicely. The best way to stay motivated is TO SEE RESULTS and you will begin to see them within 6 to 8 weeks. It is these results that will talk back to your negative self doubts, and force them to see that they are wrong about you. The trick is to stick with something long enough to A: get past those feelings of discomfort against the changes you are making, and B: to begin to see results that will in and of themselves provide you with positive reinforcement and further motivation.

To get these results, include cardiovascular activity at 50 to 60 per cent of your max heart rate (charts are available online) for 20 minutes or longer — and do those activities 4 to 5 times a week. Work up by trying it twice the first week, three times the second, and so on, until you feel challenged but are still recovering in between sessions. Once you feel you are getting the hang of it, up the intensity to 60 to 70 per cent of your max heart rate.

If you are new to fitness, see a doctor and have him or her clear you for whatever activity you would like to try. Pick your activity by thinking back to your school days: what sports did you enjoy? Was basketball super fun? Did you play hockey? Were you on the track and field team? Have you ever tried a step class or Zumba? Think about times when you were active and felt real joy or fun. These are the activities you can begin to practice.

If you try something three or more times and truly hate it, switch to something else until you hit something that resonates with you. I am a runner. Bikers hate running, walkers hate biking, hikers hate treadmills, etc etc. go with what feels good and you will keep doing it.

The most simple starting point is walking — start flat, then walk faster, then add hills, then switch to two minutes slow running and two minutes walking, then up to five minutes slow running to one minute walking, and on and on. Slap on some headphones and listen to music to make it fun, or bring a buddy along.

I remember reading a post on social media not long ago — it was a woman who had taken a picture of herself giving the finger to the camera — the post read something like — "I f*&king hate running!" And went on to list all the reasons she was hating it. I found this posting quite baffling …. If you start doing something and don't like it, then switch to something else. Don't try to force yourself to continue an activity you hate just because it's the first thing you tried, or your friends are doing it — or whatever the reason. I replied to this woman's post and in a gentle way, suggested she try something else. I still chuckle a bit when I think about someone posting negative comments and rude pictures on a running group with thousands of members — to me it advertised what so many of us do in our lives — we continue struggling along when something isn't working, instead of just trying to change the program to something we may actually like and feel better about.

Once you have picked something and started doing it, use all of your mental powers and make an agreement with yourself to stick to it for at least a month — count 30 days on the calendar and cross off every day after you have done your activity that day. Say out loud to yourself each morning: "Today is day X" This creates visual motivation and also talks back to that pesky subconscious devil on your shoulder trying to make your quit. Within a couple of weeks — if you keep at it — you will begin to see some of what I call "early signs of success" - I want you to pay attention to these signs and to note them and congratulate yourself when you begin to notice these signs. These signs are powerful motivators that let you know that you are on the right track.

Early signs your walking/running/biking program is working

1. You start to feel elation while you are working out

2. You get out of breathe a little less each day

3. Some of your clothing may get a bit looser

4. You sleep better/wake up with more energy

5. People at work notice that you look different and tell you so

6. You go a little further and a little faster each day

7. You begin to think you can actually do this

The reason why it's important to note these signs is that they are subtle enough to ignore, but powerful indeed when focussed upon. And what you need to do in the early stages of any fitness program is to focus on each and every positive sign you notice, no matter how small or insignificant it may seem. This is what I mean when I say over and over that conditioning your mind is just as important as conditioning your body.

If during the early stages of your fitness program, you just bemoan the negative things such as not being able to eat junk food or feeling sore from working out, then you are really giving your subconscious mind ammunition with which to attack you with. By this I mean those feelings of fear, anxiety and discomfort that you will surely feel as you embark upon a program that involves very profound change. It is hard enough to fight back against the negative interruptions your mind will throw up at you to try to get you back into your comfortable old routine. If, on top of this, you are consciously complaining and allowing negative thoughts and words to clutter your conscious mind, you will honestly be doomed to failure.

So do yourself a huge favour and look for all the little positives that are happening in your life — comment on them — think about them in a way that is joyful and grateful — talk about the positive changes you are experiencing to others around you and allow them to help you by encouraging you, which they will surely do. If I had to say it in one sentence, pretend that your job is to be a cheerleader to yourself, and cheerlead yourself the same way you would your very best friend who was going through the exact same thing.

Another very helpful and powerful motivational tool that thousands of people benefit from is creating a visual chart or list that can powerfully motivate you. This is an exercise in Cognitive Behavioural Therapy, which is a powerful method used to identify your limiting beliefs and to reframe those beliefs into something positive.

Take a piece of paper and make two columns. Title Column A "Benefits of being overweight and sedentary" and title Column B "Disadvantages of being overweight and sedentary." Take your time with each column and really try to find benefits to your current situation as well as disadvantages. I asked a friend of mine in this situation to do a sample of the form and here's what hers looked like:

Advantages to OW

* I never have to exercise.

* I can eat whatever I want

* People feel sorry for me

* I can watch TV every night

Disadvantages

* I feel bad about myself

* I don't like my body

* I feel depressed about life

* I feel physically limited/unwell

* I don't feel sexy or desirable

* I worry a lot about my health

* jealous of fit, attractive women

* I hate pictures of myself

* I worry about my health

* It seems like I'll never succeed

A few things may surprise you about this list for yourself. First off, you may be surprised that there are some advantages to staying the way you are. When you really think about it, it's easier in some ways to stay inactive and overweight. You can watch TV every night, eat as much ice cream as you want, never have to feel the pain of sore muscles and basically just keep everything comfortable and the same in your life.

BUT ... You will never have the body you deserve and want, you will never rock that bikini, you won't enjoy the fantastic feeling of smashing your life goals, you won't be able to take photos of yourself and feel great posting them, you won't have the pleasure of knowing your blood pressure is back to normal and your joint pain has vanished; you won't see your muscle tone; you won't feel how sexy and desirable your body is; you will never be the person that you really want to be.

After you make this list, post it on the fridge in plain sight, and use it as a daily reminder and motivator — add more items to each column as you think of them. Writing down your thoughts has a very powerful impact on your mind — it allows you to take a focussed look at your own thoughts — to view them objectively on paper. Writing things down frankly helps you learn a lot about yourself, and you will be amazed how much is going on inside your brain that you really didn't know about.

Honestly, you can read books like this one until the cows come home, but the way you know you are doing great is by seeing results. It's a good idea to tune into the signs of results (that do not include a number on a scale): mainly that you are feeling better about yourself, and you are finding the joy in activity again!

Personal trainers like me can help and motivate, teach and train, and really care about their clients. But for those of you practicing self-sabotage, it may not give you results if you aren't ready to truly make changes.

There is something powerful about writing things down and reviewing them. You may think that you know your thoughts, but you actually don't know many of the unconscious decisions that you make every day. You don't really know what things you are attracting to yourself because there is a part of your mind that believes them to be true.

Here's an example of how your subconscious mind makes decisions for you faster than your conscious mind can. You are emptying out your dishwasher and you pull out the container that holds your utensils and put it on the counter in front of you — you automatically start grabbing forks — out of all the cutlery you suddenly see only forks and your hands reach out and grab forks, ignoring the knives and spoons, etc. You are doing this so automatically that your conscious mind could not keep up, even if it wanted to. Next, you move onto knives and do the same thing — your hands just reach for knife after knife, without you even having to think about it.

Or think about driving to work in the morning — your subconscious mind guides you as you put the key into the ignition, fire up the car, put it into drive then take off. You probably do this in the morning and drive to work, all while your conscious mind thinks about something else.

The point I am making is that we are all picking out the things that are going to happen to us next, kind of like being on autopilot. Your autopilot right now might be to get in the car after work, drive home, collapse on the couch and turn on the television — zone out for an hour, then get up and make dinner, do a clean up and collapse on the couch again feeling exhausted by your efforts, thinking you could not possibly do anything more. These decisions feel like they are conscious, but in reality, you are continuing on with routines that are so well established in your subconscious mind that they are controlling 97 per cent of your life without you really even making the conscious choice anymore. And to be honest and direct, nothing WILL change until you step up and change your own mental programming.

This can be done, it just takes some internal work along with some external commitment. If you do nothing else, then at least attempt to follow the advice in the next chapter and take on three new positive habits into your life. The great thing about positive habits is that they can, with time, cancel out negative habits and have the added benefit of being good for you and for your self esteem.

Chapter 6
The Trinity: Meditation, Exercise, Journaling

When Post Traumatic Stress led me to seek counselling a few years ago, I was introduced to some pretty interesting information about the human brain by a skilled counsellor. When we suffer a trauma, our brains get caught in an endless loop of re-living the bad event or events that happened to us — and this can go on for years in the form or regular flashbacks and feelings of fear and doom that can be paralyzing and bring us back to feeling as if the incident were going on right in front of us again in the moment, instead of being safely in the past where it belongs.

Think of this as your monkey brain caught in the fight or flight cycle, making you always feel angry or frustrated or scared. This was happening to me and it was robbing me of sleep, causing me to feel extreme fear about a past event, and making me feel powerless over my circumstances. Without help, I'm not sure what would have become of me. My counsellor explained to me that while coming to a full recovery takes time and work with a professional, there are three things that are crucial to getting over any trauma that pretty much everyone can do and cost little or no money: namely journaling, meditation and exercise.

Wow. Did you ever imagine that you could begin the work on healing yourself by just using these three tools regularly? And isn't it great to know that exercise cannot only change your body, but can, more importantly, help heal past trauma?

I began meditating right away and I have never looked back. That was five years ago. I was one of those people who thought there was no time in the day for something like meditation and I really didn't see the point in it. I was totally caught up in a do, do, do mentality. Stopping myself and being still? These were completely foreign concepts to me!

What did meditation have to do with the fact that I had suffered through a traumatic experience? It certainly wasn't going to make everything better, that wasn't possible, I thought. But I was wrong. Meditation helped me to get control over the present moment, which in turn helped me make better decisions which went on to literally help me get my life back on track in a way it had never been before. It was a fundamental shift.

Fast forward to present day, and I would think a day to be very poor indeed if it did not start with at least 20 minutes of any form of meditation. Meditation slows down the mind and the body and helps us be in the present moment and become the observer of our thoughts. The present moment is all we have — ever. In concentrating during meditation, we can find a quiet place inside our minds where answers live to virtually all of our problems.

Practice a beginning meditation:

Try to set aside just five to ten minutes a day to start with. Pick a quiet, warm spot in a dark room where you can sit or lie comfortably but not fall asleep. If you meditate at the same time in the same place every day, you will find it gets easier and easier to relax and let go. Being warm, in darkness and in quiet are the best circumstances in which to start your meditation, so try to carve out a small place in your home where you are able to get this.

Close your eyes and begin to simply pay attention to your breath — breathe in and out slowly at least five times, paying close attention to how your body takes the air in, and then releases it. Pay attention to the very brief pause between you inhalation and exhalation. Listen to the sound of your breathing and feel how it feels different to breathe in, and to breathe out. Thoughts will be coming and going from your mind — let them — think of them as clouds in the sky that is your mind. Let them float in and out and float away, not attaching yourself to any or making any of them into worries.

If you are new to meditation, try a body scan for the first few weeks. After about five minutes of deep breathing and paying very close attention to your breathe, start at the top of your head and begin focusing on one part of your body at a time, moving from top to bottom. Feel your scalp, then your face, your neck, your shoulders, your arms, your torso, your upper legs, your lower legs and your feet. As you concentrate on each part of your body, keep you focus on it until you feel it tingling and burning, softening and relaxing. This type of body scan is very good at relaxing the body, and help open up the mind to suggestions.

Next, try using a mantra or affirmation to steady your mind onto a positive course. A very powerful and simple one is: "I am whole, perfect, strong, powerful, loving, harmonious and happy." Try repeating a few I am affirmations in your mind as you breathe in and out and try to keep your body soft and relaxed.

Affirmations may seem silly to some people (especially after SNL made fun of them so much), but the fact is that they work, and they work very well. Although you may not believe them at first, the trick with an affirmation, like the trick to any success in life, is to keep doing it and to not give up, no matter how discouraged you may feel at times. After a while, affirmations will get under your skin, and then they will begin to penetrate your subconscious mind. All your subconscious mind does is run programs that it has learned to run based on the experiences you have had and your reactions to those experiences. But like any computer, it can be re-programmed. And for many of us, we require new programming because our current data is outdated: it served a certain purpose at a certain time in our lives.

For example, when you were 11 and felt scared and alone because you may have been bullied at school or perhaps treated badly at home, you may have snuck into your bedroom at night and comforted yourself with food, or just with crying and feeling bad or anxious. I know how this feels because I have been there myself. These behaviours served you as a child because you had limited power and limited ability to cope because you were a child living with a family you did not choose, and also because your emotional intelligence was still developing. The very unfortunate thing about our developing years is that, unless our parents do a perfect job and our schooling is completely positive, we are going to be left with some emotional hangovers. And let's face it: hardly any of us had it perfect growing up. The vast majority of us had challenges, and we had to develop coping skills to deal with them as children. But nobody explained to us that when we grew up, it would be helpful to reprogram our minds, because those coping skills that helped us as children are oftentimes actually harmful to us as adults.

Here's a personal example: When I was a child, I got very scared before going to bed at night. I would hear news stories on the television and become very afraid of people getting hurt or flooding or even killer bees coming and killing us. I would get terrible stomach aches and my mother, not know what was wrong, would give me Bromoseltzer, thinking there was something physically wrong with me. The stomach aches and butterflies were, of course, anxiety. I was a sensitive child and news stories frightened me — no one explained to me what anxiety was, or how to deal with it. I also had things happen in my home that were scary, which added to my anxiety. By the time I grew up, I was a heavily anxious person. Any kind of stress — like a crowded airport, or doing something wrong at work, or feeling like I had offended someone, or thinking something I had done could cause someone to get hurt or injured — would send me into a tailspin and the symptoms were very physical and very real — heart palpitations, stomach aches, tight chest, hyperventilations, feeling faint, even full on panic attacks.

But think about it — these feelings all occurred over things that were really just every day occurrences that most people wouldn't flicker an eyelid over. But because I was programmed to be fearful and didn't know why, I just keep over reacting to things this way well into my 30s. Once I finally began meditating, I also began re-programming some of that internal conflict with positive messages. The thing about positives and negatives is that both cannot exist as thoughts in your mind at the same time. In other works, if you simply focus on replacing a negative thought with a positive one and guard your thoughts as much as possible, then your mind will not get carried away down the rabbit hole. And in life, it is much easier to make better choices for yourself and your life when you are thinking positive thoughts and not letting your old negative patterns carry you away on the worry train of life.

Journaling, which goes hand in hand with meditation, allows us to get out our most hidden fears and thoughts — and once we read them over — we are able to distance ourselves from then. This helps us gain back control over what our thoughts are. Writing things out helps our conscious mind see when our subconscious mind is trying to pull the wool over our eyes.

For example, you may write down some thoughts and read them later and see that you wrote that you never succeeded at anything and would always be a failure. Then your more reasonable conscious mind might say, actually that isn't true at all, I've succeeded at lots of jobs, and in this and that relationship, plus these projects and those proposals. When this happens you can go back and confirm that the limiting beliefs you had about yourself are actually 100% FALSE. Maybe you wrote that, "I will never be thin" when in fact, you are only human and cannot see the future therefore this believe is completely false. Then you might go back and write something a little more true beside the false statement that says something like, "I have not yet had the chance to be skinny but lots of people lose significant amounts of weight and become thin and there isn't any reason why I couldn't be one of them!" Poof! Just like that you have journaled your way through a statement that may have been holding you back for much of your adult life. This is powerful.

Number three after meditation and journaling to combat trauma, but certainly not last, is exercise. Exercise has too many heath benefits to name but lets just list off a few:

* Improves cardiovascular health, which in turn decreases your chance of having a heart attack or stroke

* Helps promote weight loss, and can keep you feeling good about yourself emotionally

* Improves flexibility and range of movement — as you age — being flexible and able to move WILL separate you from those who are not physical — and are far more prone to injuries and falls due to lack of physical strength, flexibility and agility, which all help you in situations such as walking on an icy path, stumbling over a curb, having to jump out of the way of a moving object, etc

* Decreases your interest in self-harming behaviours such as heavy drinking, smoking, binge eating, poor self image and self talk and low self esteem

* Increases self esteem by helping you to feel better about your body and about the choices you are making and feeling in control of your life

* Decreases chance of age-related high blood pressure, certain types of diabetes, decreased bone density,

muscle atrophy, etc. and certain types of cancers and slows down the aging process, helping to prevent fragility and injuries

* Can improve mood and outlook on life and help with a better general sense of happiness and well-being.

* Makes you a positive role model for your children, spouse, brothers and sisters, co-workers and friends

* Allows you to remain able-bodied and confident to participate in a wide range of hobbies and activities, from skiing and hiking to traveling and exploring

Exercise, to be frank, is about the closest thing to the Fountain of Youth that we as human beings have. It is something we can do for ourselves that puts us in the driver's seat. We get to control how much we do, what we do, when we do it and how we do it. We can take back control over our bodies and at the same time, our minds.

When we lose control of our bodies, we feel like we are losing control over our lives, and in a sense, we are. Once you gain a certain amount of excess weight, it begins to affect other parts of your life. Think about it. For one thing, the less activity you do, the less you want to do, and the less you are able to do. The vicious cycle will cause you to continue gaining weight unless you stop the slide.

When your body begins to take on a shape that is not pleasing to you, you also begin to feel self conscious about yourself. It affects how you feel being naked, either alone or with your partner. It also causes you to begin to lose some of your self-esteem, which again can lead to a downward spiral which can make you feel worse about yourself.

Feeling bad about yourself in turn can cause a lot more negative thoughts to start cropping up in your mind, and if they are not replaced by positive ones right away, they can begin to affect your overall sense of happiness and worth. These in turn can lead to more severe problems like anxiety and depression. Not to be gloom and doom, not everyone who gains weight is going to be or feel unhappy, but it is a contributing factor to many people's negative feelings about themselves.

On the other hand, if you do keep your body in good shape and remain active, it's just one more tool in your self-esteem toolkit that you can count on each and every day. And the more you exercise and feel better about yourself, the more you WANT to exercise and feel better about yourself. Make it through the first 30 days of an exercise program, and I can almost guarantee you that you will not stop, because you will not want to stop.

This is a very good time to talk about momentum. Momentum is defined as the impetus and driving force gained by the development of a process or course of events — it is a state of being or doing during which things begin to move along as if they are somehow powering themselves, instead of being forced or pushed along.

Momentum is something we have all felt or experienced. Think about something as simple as riding a bike — it's a bit of labour to get on and start pedalling while maintaining your balance and peddling through the first few rotations. But soon enough, you are moving along at a good clip and the effort (on relatively flat roads) feels minimal. Momentum does not happen immediately, because it is usually the product of the introduction of some force or power that, "Gets you going."

This is a great metaphor for your journey towards becoming active, losing fat and gaining muscle, becoming fit, and living a happier and healthier life. If you think of the process of getting fit in terms of momentum, it will help you greatly by providing you with some mental support, which is even more important than the physical act of working out. Without your mind and thoughts supporting your actions, you are far more likely to fail and go back to your old ways. So regarding momentum you need to know and believe deeply that the beginning of this process — this first 30 days — may feel difficult at first — uncomfortable and even unpleasant, because of your subconscious mind trying to trick you into stopping. This is very much the same as getting on the bike and starting to try to peddle and balance and get going all at the same time. It feels hard in the beginning, but if you just commit to sticking it out, then sometime during that first 30 days, you will feel momentum start to kick in. Your body will get used to motion and want to stay in motion and feel better and better while in motion, just like it feels better and better as you get going on that bicycle. Momentum also brings with it feelings of elation and of wanting to keep going, and not stop. Once you start to gain momentum, you will see your accomplishments go up dramatically, while your discomfort goes down dramatically. Once you get really into the momentum phase of your fitness routine, I guarantee you there will be no stopping you. So understand and plan for momentum to kick it. Know that it will and believe that it will. And know that it will feel great when it does kick in.

Chapter 7

Work Sucks your Energy, but it Doesn't Have to

Ok, let's just say you are on board with me so far. You have begun doing some meditation and journaling, you have identified some limiting self-beliefs and are working to refute them. You have embarked on the very beginnings of a health and fitness plan. You are thinking, where the heck do I start? Let's spend a few chapters talking about some practical nuts and bolts of getting you motivated and on a personalized fitness plan.

First, let's talk about the place you spend most of your waking hours: your job!

What does my fitness have to do with my job??? The answer: plenty! How you take care of yourself during your workday will do one of two things: have you ending the day feeling mentally and physically exhausted and unable to muster up the energy for a walk, run or workout; or allow you to finish the day with close to your full energy potential in tact, meaning you feel more like going to the gym — you feel like you have the energy and you aren't fighting pain and fatigue.

Listen: as a certified ergonomics technician for the government, part of my work duties includes assessing individuals in an office setting and determining what they are doing incorrectly that can and often is exacerbating certain muscular skeletal conditions, and to provide generally easy to implement tips and changes that can miraculously transform mood, energy and morale in the workplace.

Let's look at this like a graph and assume that many of the people who are reading this book work in an office setting, or spend at least part of the day sitting at a desk or workstation.

On Monday morning at 8:30 a.m. you walk into the doors to work — you had a relaxing weekend, went on some nice walks, ran, worked out at the gym, slept well and also spent some down time just cooking, relaxing and making some nice meals with your partner. Let's say, for the sake of argument, that you are not ill or suffering any pain that morning — you are at 100 per cent physical and mental efficiency.

The morning starts going and you hunker down — you're busy! You don't get up from your computer once before 10 a.m., and then you forget all about taking your 15 minute break. You are starting to feel tired, despite the several cups of coffee you have drunk to try and "kick start" your dreary Monday morning. Your neck muscles are starting to tense up and your right wrist is starting to ache, but you tell yourself you are too busy to take a break and you just soldier on.

By 11 a.m. your efficiency level has dropped to about 75 per cent of what you had when you walked through the doors, but you've been working so hard that you are not present enough in your body to even notice this shift downwards.

Your next mistake is to skip going out for a walk on your lunch break and instead eating a sandwich and have another cup of coffee at your desk while continuing to work or, worse, driving somewhere and eating a heavy lunch at a restaurant, stuffing yourself, then driving back to work.

After lunch you feel tired and drained — as if you could fall asleep on your desk — because you have had no real break, no fresh air, and zero exercise. You tell yourself it's just the lunch you ate making you feel tired. It's not. You have now beat down your own efficiency level to about 45 per cent and you are continuing on a downward slide. Your muscles are cramped and stiff, your oxygen levels are depleted and your eyes are strained.

Somehow you keep going, and tell yourself to "power through" because it's 3 p.m. and you have to get X, Y and Z done before 4:30 p.m. (why, is the apocalypse coming? Is it your very last day of work?? What's the emergency anyway?) — So you skip your afternoon break or go to the coffee room and grab a drink … pounding back more coffee and not moving around and not getting any fresh air and oxygen to your brain.

So guess what happens to you when the bell rings at 4:30 or 5 p.m. and your work day is finally done? You walk out the door and tromp down the steps to the parking lot and think to yourself: "OH God, I feel like a pile of crap! I can't possibly go to the gym. I'm exhausted. I need to go home and lie down for a while then maybe I'll feel like getting out." Here's the bad news — no, you likely won't feel like going out for that run or that walk after you go home and lie down.

Why?

Because by the end of your long and productive day, you had dwindled down your efficiency from 100 per cent at the beginning of the day down to somewhere around 20 to 25 per cent by the end. And the result is that you feel sluggish and tired, sapped of energy and lacking ambition to do anything fun or physical. Try to remember though, reading back over this sad little Monday tale — that you actually did this to yourself. You did this to yourself by not implementing a few simple self-care techniques that are proven to greatly reduce these energy losses over a day, and turn this story around.

So let's rewind this fable back to Monday morning at 8:30 a.m. after the same fun and relaxing weekend and see you, as a person who cares about yourself and loves yourself, could have done differently.

This time around, you take a short break every 20 minutes to half hour starting right from 9 a.m. — you get up out of your chair and do a bit of walking, you roll your shoulders back a number of times, which you notice feels good — it feels good because it is the opposite movement to being hunkered down over a keyboard and computer monitor. You even do some reverse arm rolls — feeling the blood flowing through your body.

You also practice good eye hygiene by taking your focus away from the close up monitor and gazing out the nearest window for a minute or to — looking out at some nature or at least a tree and some birds — and taking a few deep breaths. Honestly, it only takes about 1 to 2 minutes to take a little mini break like this. Let's say you take at least 2 of them before your coffee — then during coffee you take a short walk around the block and take the stairs back up and not the elevator — you breathe in fresh air and get your heart pumping for 15 minutes. Low and behold, it's now 10:30 a.m. and you are still close to 100 per cent efficiency — this scenario is factually based and is based on large scale studies.

Carrying on with our new Monday scenario, you take a half hour walk outside at lunch — briskly and out in the fresh air, and continue taking mini breaks every half hour or so during the work day, then take a second 15 minute break during which you go out on the deck and do a few jumping jacks, squats and march on the spot and drink a big glass of water.

Now here we are at the end of the same day — but this time you have retained 75 to 85 per cent of your daily efficiency. Today, you feel that you have the energy to go for a brisk walk, and maybe even hit the gym for 20 minutes.

The reason why this chapter is so important to any book on changing your fitness habits is that many, many of us skip self-care techniques during the workday, because we think that we have to work without breaks to get things done. This simply isn't true. If we treat ourselves with care and respect all day long at work, we will have so much more to give back to ourselves after work, and so much more for our loved ones. If you want to make fitness a part of your life, one good way to start is to ensure that you don't have that, "I feel wasted" feeling at the end of any workday.

Chapter 8

Think how Winners Think

Whether we are talking about a goal to get a great job, make a certain amount of money, meet the right partner, or become fit and healthy — winners all have the same thing in common — they believe in themselves. No matter what happens to them; no matter if they fail at something the first or second or even tenth try; and no matter what stands in their way, they believe in themselves. This is neither luck nor chance. We know this is true because winners have come from every socio-economic level and every kind of background. The only advantage that one human being can have over another is that they were either raised up in a supportive environment and find believing in themselves comes naturally, or they learned through single-minded effort that any goal they could dream of, they could achieve.

Winners set goals for themselves and they work hard to attain them. They also continually re-evaluate their goals which helps them to know when they can be ticked off the list, or when a new or higher goal can be added.

The first thing a trainer would ask you before even beginning to consider what type of program to put you on is: what are your fitness goals?

As you really begin to start moving — start doing your daily walks, or walks/runs for 30 to 45 minutes at least 5 days a week — spend a bit of time working on your fitness goals. Here are a few things to consider and keep in mind when making up your list of goals.

First and foremost, try and make your short-term goals such that you are fairly sure you can attain them — the point is that once you crush that first goal, you will be extremely happy with yourself and ready to set a new goal that may have seemed unattainable to you two months before. For example, if you are 60 lbs over your weight when you were at your fittest 15 years ago, try a goal of losing 8 lbs over the first month. How would that feel?

Now make notes of how you are going to do that. I am going to lose 8 lbs in two months. To do this, I am going to walk/run three to four days a week for at least 30 minutes. I am also going to research a low-fat, healthy meal plan and make an agreement with myself and my family to stick to it. I am going to start drinking water throughout the day, especially when I feel like I might want to cheat on my meal plan. I am also going to try at least one class per week at my local gym, and when I find one I like, I am going to try and go one or two times a week. When I am out walking I am going to focus on working to a medium intensity level, so that I elevate my heart rate and warm up my body and burn calories.

After the first couple of weeks, I will check on my progress — if I am losing weight at about the rate of one to two lbs a week, I will keep going while slowly increasing the time and intensity of my workouts to match my fitness level. If I am not making progress, I will take a good hard look at my diet and my exercise program, and make some adjustments that I think will help me get on the right track.

Try to read your goal daily and really, really try to stick to it. The magic about goals is that writing them down really does help make them happen, and I know it's an almost guaranteed path to success.

One problem that some women in particular run into is that they have some success with their fitness program, but they get discouraged after achieving so much because they are stuck on a number or a way they want to look that is unrealistic. Let's face it, none of us are going to look like we did when we were 23 at 45. I consider myself to be in very good shape - FOR MY AGE - but I see gals at the gym half my age and know they could kick my butt from here to the other side of the moon. But I can run 10 km and not be sore, I can work out at the gym six days a week and have the energy to do so, I have good muscle tone, low body fat, high bone density, good hydration levels and have a slim build based on my many years of running.

I have friends who get depressed and frustrated because they long to shed that last 10 or 15 lbs so they can be at a certain number on the scale. They don't accept that their bodies have changed, especially after having children, or even simply from the process of aging. When women come to me about his, I honestly say, "You look great! And you sure don't look like you need to lose that much more weight." Then I will usually ask them about their routine. If they are working out at least four times a week and maintaining a healthy diet and they look fit, seem fit, feel fit and have the kind of vitality that non-fit people cannot fake, then I will often say, "Why not take it easy on yourself and maybe re-think that final goal. You look amazing to me — focus on that for a while, and see how you feel in a month or two."

It's a sad thing to me when someone comes so far and accomplishes so much, but then gets stuck on an ideal of perfection that they can't reach and can't shake. It can actually completely derail people. Keep your goals in line with what is realistic for your age, health, body type and self esteem. And again, talk to and treat yourself the same way you would a friend that you truly loved and cared about. It will make all the difference in the world.

On a final note, I am not trying to say you can't reach big goals — there are many people who do lose 100 or more lbs and they do it one step, one class, one meal, at a time. But they also had to start with realistic goals. Walk to the end of the block, then two blocks, then a mile, then five. In fact, one could say that the way to achieve goals that today seem like a star's distance away, is by setting little goals that slowly, but steadily, lead you towards that star. Then after a while you think, "MMM, I used to think that star was so far away, but now I can see it is almost within my grasp!"

Remember: becoming a winner is a lot easier if you think about realistic goals, write them down, take steps to follow them, then update them regularly to adapt to your progress and where you would like to go next.

Chapter 9

Bad Habits Reflect How you Feel About Yourself

Ok, you've decided to get fit — you have started walking three to four times a week for 45 minutes, and added some classes — you're awesome! You have made it through the first couple of weeks and you are starting to see changes — while you are working on these fantastic changes - Now is a good time to start looking at dropping any bad habits that you have picked up along your life journey — particularly the ones that you just know are not helping you towards your goal of becoming a fit and healthy person: mentally, physically, emotionally and spiritually.

Habits are really interesting because they are something we picked up — often in childhood or early adulthood — that served a purpose in our early years. However, often we hold onto bad habits throughout our lives because, well frankly it's easy, and we don't question why we are continuing the behaviour. Again, this is a trick of the subconscious mind. Because we perform certain rituals and behaviours completely on autopilot, we might be stuck with them our whole lives unless we are will to bring them to the forefront and expend some effort changing them.

Here's a few examples, many of which I have dealt with as my own personal demons — some I've completely overcome, some I am working on, and others I know are long-term projects.

Smoking and Drinking: the kings of the bad habit hill

Oh, how I used to love smoking and drinking, and drinking and smoking! Even as a runner and weight lifter, I went through a phase during which I was drinking wine and smoking cigarettes daily. Both are incredibly stupid habits for a fit person to have, but I used to rationalize it by joking that my good side and my bad side were fighting each other, and that I just wasn't sure yet who was going to win. Little did I know how true that statement was! Of course the problem with this kind of behaviour is that it will eventually come back and bite you right in the ass! A cancer diagnosis, a heart attack, a stroke — you flirt with these every year that you continue smoking and drinking to excess.

After about six months of seeing a good therapist and really being attentive to how cigarettes were affecting me and tapering off my smoking, I was able to pick a quit day and stick to it. I have, to be fair, had to quit smoking a couple of times in my life. I know it is hard. Get whatever help you need and keep trying to quit. Honestly, you really cannot call yourself a healthy person if you work out and smoke, not to mention the fact that you greatly increase your chances of many preventable illnesses.

Quitting smoking while you are working on becoming fit may seem a lot to handle, but actually the two really compliment each other and help you build your confidence and self-esteem. The less you smoke the more you want to work out and the more you work out, the less you want to smoke — try it!

My husband recently quit smoking after forty years as a smoker. He remembers sneaking puffs off his grandpa's pipe while sitting on the old man's knee when he was just a small boy. I love him dearly, but I honestly did not believe that he would be able to quit. He actually would pull the filters off each cigarette and smoke them straight — that's how tobacco addicted he was. When he picked the same week to quit as the week he planned to start going back to karate again, I was even more skeptical. I thought he was trying to take on way too much, too soon. However, here it is six months later and he is still not smoking and still going to karate and currently in better shape than most men his age. I am very proud of him. If you ask him why he succeeded he would say that he was completely mentally prepared to quit and had been doing work on his emotional well-being for several years in preparation for making these last two big changes. So anything is possible if you believe in yourself and guard your thoughts against any little voices that try to derail you.

Similarly with drinking — while I don't know that I will ever give up wine completely (I'm Italian, after all), I stopped drinking at all during the work week a long while ago. It started out as an experiment — because I wasn't totally sure I could do it — and I thought to myself that if I could not manage to reduce my drinking, than I would have to look at stopping altogether for the good of my health. I just did not like myself when I was needing that glass of wine to unwind after a long day almost every day. Honestly, it feels great saving wine for weekends and special occasions, not to mention all those saved calories! Light to moderate drinking is generally not thought to be harmful, but again if you reduce drinking when you start exercising the two good habits will help you stay on track and move you towards your goals quickly.

Working out without putting in the effort: This is an awful habit that I see in the gym daily! Please, if you do this, stop immediately! Do NOT read a magazine or book while working out; do NOT lean on cardio machines as if your life depended on it; do NOT talk more than you work out; do NOT daydream or text on your phone; simply put, do NOT fool around or be unfocussed while working out! When you are working out, be 100 per cent focused and put all of your attention, effort and energy into what you are doing. Anything less is about as good as not being there at all. Crappy workouts are one of the worst habits you can develop, so don't start it and if you have that habit — please — drop it immediately. Honestly, this is the reason people 'work out' for a few weeks then quit because they weren't getting results. In reality, they were texting, flipping through magazines while slowing peddling an exercise bike, or just not putting in the effort required to achieve results. You will only get out of exercise what you put in — it's an exact equation.

Watching too much Television/Entertainment as a hobby. Ok, hate me if you want, but television is crap. There is very little on television that is truly useful, intelligent and helpful to us in our daily lives. Most people sit around watching reality shows and sitcoms and nothing good can come into your life from spending time that way — not a blessed thing! If you care about yourself, your body and your brain, then start minimizing the amount of television you watch today. There are about a million healthier things you can do with your evening and I'll just name a few: go for a long walk outside, go to the gym and lift weights, go for a hike in the woods, go to a fitness or yoga class, call up a friend and see how they are doing, read a really good book, take your kids and dog on a little stroll and visit your neighbours, do some vigorous house cleaning or organizing, have a long hot bath, meditate or listen to binaural beats or relaxation music, have a romantic dinner and bedroom fun with your partner, do some journaling, write down some good short and long term goals, engage in any hobby that you enjoy from knitting to napping …. you get the picture. Don't just take it from me, ask anyone you know who is very fit and committed to a healthy lifestyle and I can almost guarantee you that they watch little or no television.

Using silly excuses to blow off your workouts. Honestly, once you start this nasty habit of blowing off exercising for make-believe reasons, you will continue doing so and you will not reach your fitness goals. By silly excuses I mean excuses that most of us who prioritize fitness will not use to blow off a workout — these may include feeling tired, not having enough time, having your period, feeling bloated — these are all not good enough, sorry. Good excuses for not working out include: injuries that impair your movement, being burnt out after working out hard for a number of days in a row and needing rest, illnesses that cannot be helped by working out like fevers, flus, respiratory illness, etc and simply being too damn sore from the workout you did the day before or two days before.

There are many other bad habits I could list out here but ultimately, if we are honest with ourselves we know what our bad habits are. Try to think about tackling some of them during the time when you begin your work out routine — try to maintain your good new habits and shun your old ones for just three weeks, then see how you feel. I can promise you that if you give yourself a fighting chance, you will permanently drop many of your bad habits or at least reduce their hold on you, while at the same time gaining confidence in your ability to become who you really are; fit, healthy and happy!

Chapter 10

Never Fail Again

There are many reasons why people fail time and time again in their efforts to get fit. Having worked out at gyms for many years, worked in an office environment for just as many years, and having learned the real scientific formula to successful weight loss in studying to become a Certified Personal Trainer, it is clear what stumbling blocks people face that hold them back from becoming fit. Here are a few of them — can you pick out the ones that relate to you?

The roller coaster dieter/exerciser

I know many office workers who fall into this category. They start a fitness program and strict diet regime, and often try to force their spouses into getting on board (bad idea). They manage to stay on track for a couple of weeks, then, after the first unexpected binge, or overindulgence at a party, instead of getting back on track, they just give up entirely and go back to feeling bad about themselves and give up exercising and watching calories. A few weeks later when they dare to get back on the scale and get frightened by the rising figure, they jump back on that strict wagon — only to fall off it again — yes, about two weeks later.

These are interesting cases — they often know what they need to do and are capable of doing it — many can easily plan a decent workout routine and diet all on their own, without consulting a trainer. So what goes wrong every single time?

In short, they don't believe in themselves and they are afraid to give up the comfortable routine that keeps their lives on autopilot. Honestly, if this is you, you may want to consider seeing a counsellor before you plan your next get fit plan. Talk to someone you trust about what your real fears are: that you will never be fit? That you are afraid to fail? That there is a voice in you that says you will always be fat? That there is a voice inside you that says, "You are a loser?" These voices inside our heads are insidious and many of us have beliefs about ourselves that are very negative at the core. This can affect many parts of our lives, not just our appearance.

Just when we are starting to feel good in a relationship, we might sabotage it. Just when we have landed a good job, we might do things that we know will cause us to lose it. I'm not a counsellor, but I know that I myself needed help - I sabotaged many parts of my life because of my skewed beliefs about myself. However, I am living proof that this doesn't have to be who you are. If you keep stopping yourself just before you finally begin to achieve the success you want, then it's time to get your feelings about yourself out in the open. After all, the only person getting out there and running and keeping to that meal plan — is you — no one can walk this path for you. And to walk it, you must believe in your ability to make it to the end.

The refuse to diet/refuse to exercise club

The vast majority of us work at jobs that don't allow us to achieve fitness goals during the work day. If you are fortunate enough to have a job that makes you happy and keeps you fit and active, then you have it made!

Us office folks, managers, drivers, teachers, clerks, etc etc — are not so lucky. We are forced to sit at desks in an unnatural position and we get very little opportunity to move around. After I got hired at the government job I am in now, I knew that I would need to get most of my exercise outside of the office. I began walking for a half hour every single day at lunch. That means walking in the rain, wind, snow and any other kind of crappy weather you can imagine. Walking at lunch and making as much effort to move around at work as possible usually gets me up to around 6,000 steps per work day. After work every day I run for about 30 minutes then do a 20 minute weight routine (one hour) which adds up to a pretty well rounded day. I'm home by just after 6 pm, which leaves plenty of time for making dinner, eating, and some relaxation time.

During these work days, I limit my calories because I know I am doing less to work them off. I regularly check in by weighing myself — if the scale is up, I may need to do a little more and eat a little less — if my weight drops,

I might eat a bit extra on the weekends to bump back up to normal. But you really do need both sides working together — the exercise is what raises your metabolism to assist you in burning more calories efficiently and quickly. The proper foods in reasonable portions give you the energy you need to work out — lean protein like chicken and fish, big salads, vegetables, fruit in moderation, low fat dairy and yoghurt, along with plenty of water, all compliment your exercise routine and help you to feel energized and able to work out. The best plan of action is to ensure you are getting regular physical activity 5 to 6 days per week for about an hour, while maintaining a healthy diet that limits bad fats, processed sugars, restaurant food, and large portions.

The same old, same old

One perhaps surprising reason why people don't reach their goals or give up on exercise is because they stop changing things up and do the same thing over and over again until they are so bored that they can't stand it anymore, then give up.

Change your routine up every four to six weeks — period. Keep going to the gym, just switch up your exercises. Take away one run and add in a class at the gym, ride a bike for a few weeks, then go back to running. If you go to classes, pick different ones for a few weeks and find some new favourites. Try different sports, especially during the summer months. Join a co-ed soccer team or baseball team, or take up tennis or squash.

My husband and I both got tennis rackets for about $20 each, and played one day for a laugh. Turns out, we really enjoyed it and now we play at least once a week during the late spring to fall. It's a crazy good workout and very different from running or lifting weights, which is my normal routine. It also happens to be very fun and challenging, and we have a riot doing it.

It is a fact that if you continue doing the same routine over and over again, you will stop seeing gains, and your muscles will get used to that routine, and will put out as little effort as possible to help you maintain the status quo. You will think you are in fantastic shape because you don't get sore anymore the day after your workouts. NEWSFLASH - you should be getting a bit sore regularly - DOMS (Delayed Onset Muscle Soreness) is your body's way of telling you that you are tearing little bits of your muscle fibres which is going to make them grow. You don't want to be sore every day of your life, but you should work out hard enough.

Chapter 11

Scrutinize Your Life: Where's the Rut?

Some fitness is just about fitness, and sometimes fitness is actually a reflection of what is going on in our own lives. We think that not being fit is the problem, and that if that problem were just fixed, then everything else would be perfect, right?

Not True. If you fall off the wagon, fall into a rut, dig yourself a deep hole and wallow in it — there is obviously more going on that just the fact that you have dropped your workout routine.

Sometimes we get confused about why we are not taking care of ourselves and we think that if only we lost a few pounds or felt more energy, that we would start to be happier. Honestly, sometimes our level of commitment to fitness is really just a litmus test about how our lives our going and how close to our true passion we are keeping our goals.

This reminds me of what has happened to one of my best friends over the last couple of years. Shyanne has always looked beautiful to me, but she went through a phase when she did not feel beautiful and her attempts to take up fitness were often thwarted by her full time job as a reporter, being the single mom of two busy kids, and trying to run a household in her spare time. To boot, the job was making her miserable, and her happiness level sunk to an all time low. She thought that her low energy and weight gain were the problems, but in fact they were the symptoms: the symptoms of her growing need to confront a live that just wasn't working for her any longer. Then a couple of years ago, she had the opportunity to get bought out of her job — she not only took that giant leap, but moved hundreds of miles away to start a new life in the little town where her parents lived. She wasn't exactly sure how she would make a living there, but she had some money, some support and some promising plans.

She ended up training to become a care aid for the elderly, and just excelled in the program. She instantly got a great job that she loved, and a whole new outlook on life. I hadn't seen my good friend for a couple of months, and so was excited when she came back to town for a visit. When I saw her at the store where we had agreed to meet, I almost did not recognize her! She had lost 20 lbs, her complexion was aglow and she had a beaming smile on her face. She lit up the room and I had to ask her: What did you do to change yourself so much and so quickly? Well, the long answer was doing plenty of steps at her new job (up to 18,000 per shift) and also walking on the treadmill on her breaks. She was also watching what she was eating. But when it really comes down to it, she got herself happy first, then the fitness followed. She always had a moderate diet — all she needed was to increase her activity level. She doesn't need to go to the gym, she just needs to keep doing what she is doing and maintain a sensible diet.

As you are getting serious about your fitness goals and writing them down, don't forget about the other goals you have in your life. How much are you enjoying your work? How happy are you in your current relationships? What good habits do you want to pick up? What bad habits do you need to let go?

While fitness has been a part of my life for 25 years, it was only very recently that I finally got serious about becoming a certified trainer. This in turn encouraged me to continue learning more and more about fitness, and to get the idea to write this book, a dream which at one time seemed like a very distant possibility! The point I am making, is sometimes getting fit isn't the beginning of the journey, but more like the end. Get yourself happier in the ways you can — by simply exercising your god-given right to make decisions about your own life. Once you are feeling more satisfied, more content, and more productive, you may find that starting a physical fitness program isn't something you have to try hard to do, but something you start doing because it just feels so natural and good!

Here's 7 tried and true steps you can take now if you are feeling a little confused about what to do to gain more control over your life.

1. Talk to someone — a counsellor is ideal, but even a good friend or your partner — get honest about the things in your life that are not working. I actually got a number of free sessions from a life coach who was working on her final practicum — it was so beneficial to my life and really propelled me forward. Having at least one person who is truly in your corner, listens to you and supports your goals is really key

2. Write down some goals — even ones that you might have had so many years ago that you almost forgot them — think about them — then write them down — even if they seem silly — be specific about the ones you really want to achieve — what do they look like exactly and when would you like to complete them. Write down a list of smaller short term goals (four to eight weeks out) and several long-term goals (six months to two years). Put them somewhere where you will look at them every single day. Read them, remember them - I guarantee you will start checking items off your list and that feels awesome!

3. Create a vision board and fill it with pictures of you doing what you really want to do and being who you really want to be — look at it daily — in fact many times each day — get in touch with your dreams — where you are right now and not where you have to be. Dream big!

4. Stop telling yourself you are stuck and/or have no choices — that is almost never true! You always have choices — they may seem to hard to think about —

but you could still make them if you had to. Saying you are stuck and can do nothing about it is like locking yourself up in a jail cell for life — and unless you are locked up in a jail cell for life, there is something you can do about your situation.

5. Eliminate toxic, negative people from your life or at the very least, distance yourself from them as much as possible. This may include family or others who are very close to you. But if they are constantly reinforcing negative beliefs you have about yourself, then they aren't much good for you.

6. Start doing even the smallest things towards any of your goals — if you want to learn a new skill, google some courses — you don't have to take them yet, just look at them. If you are unhappy at work maybe just prepare a new resume — you don't have to apply yet, but just get ready. If you want to start working out, go for a drive and drop in at a few gyms. Meet the owner and tour the facility — see how clean and nice it is — a lot of gyms will offer you a few days or even a week free to try their location — take advantage of this.

7. Use as many tools as you can to begin turning your negative thoughts into positive ones — apps, affirmations, goals, journaling, healing conversations, happy vision board pictures, positive self talk, self-care routines — try to capture moments when you feel good about yourself — then expand them.

Chapter 12
Believe, Do and Repeat

Get yourself ready, identify your goals in writing, get your friends and family on board, empty your cupboards of junk food, and set a date: you are ready to make that commitment to get yourself fit, healthy and active. I am going to offer you a sample for your first few months of training if you want to go for it and do so on a budget — but remember that before starting any workout program, you MUST clear it with your doctor. You must be sure you are able to start an intensive cardio program, use your muscles in their full range of motion and that your heart and lungs are healthy enough to begin exercising.

If you have clearance from your doctor and you are brand new to a workout program or you have been out of shape for a number of years and don't really know where to begin, here's a starting point.

Dietary changes

Prepare by taking all the junk food out of your home and stocking up on chicken and other lean meats, all vegetables, lots of broccoli sprouts and all kinds of salad, light dressings, pasta (I believe pasta is a healthy carb and I have never given it up), soya sauce, bananas, low fat yogurt, healthy cereals and low fat or almond milk, low fat coffee creamer, peanut butter (light or natural), white fish and salmon, and low fat granola bars and nuts such as almonds that have healthy fat.

Try to clear your space of refined sugar, potato chips, ice cream, cookies, cakes and pastries, frozen treats, chocolate bars, alcohol (wine is ok in moderation), and limit your bread intake to one servings a day at the most. These are just common sense ways to limit your fat intake. I eat a lot of fish, chicken and tons of salad at dinner every night with a yogurt salad dressing that also happens to be very low in fat. Once you start eating salad every day, you will crave it, and want to have it. Salad is super healthy for you and fills you up, along with your low-fat protein.

Stick to an easy to follow diet over the first couple of months, don't make things complicated for yourself. It's ok to drink coffee, but not more than about two cups a day. Likewise, if you want to keep drinking alcohol, one glass of wine a day most nights, maybe two on the weekends. Staying right off all or most refined sugar is best — and after a time you will stop craving it, but prepare for withdrawal systems for the first seven to 10 days.

Many people I know recently told me that the only change they made in their diet was to completely eliminate sugar and that the weight just came off! If you do decide to do this make sure you clear it with your doctor first and for the first week or two don't make any other significant dietary changes — it will be a major adjustment to your body. Recently I read a posting on social media from a young woman complaining of headaches because she had quit all sugar and coffee on the same day! I don't understand the mentality of doing this to yourself, because it simply doesn't make any sense and sets you up for instant failure, not to mention horrible physical discomfort! There are real physical withdrawal symptoms when quitting both coffee and sugar. If you are quitting sugar, give your body 10 days to adjust without making any other dietary changes.

You will know that your body has adjusted because you will suddenly go from feeling like a big pile of crap to feeling better and more energetic than before you quite eating sugar. Once you hit the good feeling stage, begin implementing other dietary changes. Refined sugar is pretty much universally believed to be one of the worst additions to the human diet. It is single handedly responsible for the onset of cavities and decay in human teeth — when it was first widely marketed in Europe people became helpless addicts to it, and rotted out their teeth. Some studies even suggest that sugar feeds cancer, and can increase your chances of contracting other types of diseases and illnesses. It doesn't have any nutritional benefits that I'm aware of. So do yourself a huge favour, and try to get as much refined sugar out of your diet as possible. Even when you reach your goal weight — as I know and believe you will — don't go back to eating refined sugar again. Or at least keep it in moderation.

Stick 100 per cent to what you plan to eat every day. If you really must cheat, don't consider it an opportunity to eat as much as you humanly can: order a dish you like and eat a moderate amount, then go back to your normal routine right after. Here is something you really need to know: most people who are at a healthy weight and are committed to a strong fitness routine generally and naturally adopt an 85 - 15 eating regime (I do this myself, just naturally). In other words, eat clean and light for 85 per cent of your meals in an average week, leaving room for more fattening favourites or treats about 15 per cent of the time. Provided you don't go insane with portions and you've worked out hard during the week, this won't derail you.

However, to get to that place, you really need to maximize your calorie deficit, or the number of calories you burn above the calories you ingest each and every day. If you want to lose a pound of fat a week, you need a 3500 calorie deficit every 7 days, or 500 calories a day. It may help you to find an app or decent web site that counts calories for you and where you can input your meals and activities for the first while. While these provide you with good guidelines, it's not an exact science.

Honestly, you need to get really active and clean up your diet, then start weighing yourself every week. If the weight is coming off, it doesn't matter worth a damn what the app says. If it isn't coming off, you may need to make more adjustments. Many factors affect how quickly or slowly people are able to lose weight, including metabolism, age, current body mass index, genetics, athletic ability, etc. The one thing common to almost all of us is that we must combine dietary changes with exercise to achieve the goal of weight loss and fitness. Doing one while ignoring the other is simply going to be a waste of your precious time on this planet.

Listen: a Fitbit will NOT make you thin! I know a woman who has had one for years and not lost a bit of weight that I can see. She bought a new one and gave away her old one after a year — as if to say that a better Fitbit would actually help her lose more weight. Kind of silly, wouldn't you say? It's kind of like what a friend of mine, Debbie, who is overweight and well aware of that fact, said to me one day. We were talking about weight loss and she was telling me how "freakishly thin" I was (haha I will always remember that), and then she said, "Have you ever seen a skinny person drinking a diet coke?" I actually thought about that and realized that, by God, nine of every ten people I have seen drinking diet coke are overweight! In the same way, I have personally noted — and I pay attention to such things — that about eight out of every ten women I see wearing fit-bits or similar gadgets are overweight and stay that way over months and years. In other words, apps and gadgets are nice to have, but it's really what's inside you — your belief in yourself and your commitment to yourself, that matters. So don't wait for a gadget or miracle device to get started. All you need is a pair of runners and a sound and prepared mind and body.

Chapter 13

Practical Fitness Routines that Work

OK, there are lots of ways to start a fitness program: you can hire a trainer, join a gym, take regular classes, join a running group, etc etc. Once you get going, you will soon develop routines that you enjoy — stick with those and explore new activities at any opportunity. What I am going to provide here is a simple sample program that requires very little expensive gear or paying a personal trainer, but can get you down the road (along with diet) to losing weight while becoming more fit. Once momentum kicks in and the good habits become instilled in you, please expand your horizons and find your zone.

Week one to four of the 30 day Cast-Away Program

Mark every day one the Calendar from day one to day 31.

Starting on day one — practice visualization and meditation exercises described earlier on in this book. After work or before, engage in a least a half hour to 40 minutes of mild to moderate cardio (walking, run/walk, biking, rowing, a class at the gym, anything that gets you moving is fine). Practice clean eating and have your last meal before 7 pm. Don't snack between meals — stick to three set meals and two healthy snacks per day. Jot down what you ate and what you did for exercise. Finish the day with a visualization exercise. Affirm your path. "I am healthy, strong and committed — getting fit it easy for me." Say this over and over all day long. If you don't believe it 100 per cent yet, that is **OK** - just keep saying it — out loud, to yourself, again and again. Spend about a half hour on youtube and bookmark some free workout sessions that look engaging to you.

The first week I would start with a minimum of three workouts that you find vigorous and challenging - Any kind of interval training, low to moderate cardio — any class you find fun, as long as it's at least 20 minutes or more. You can easily find thousands of examples on UTube, and do these workouts at home or download them onto your phone and do them at the gym if you prefer. At first you will find these workouts very hard, and you will have soreness, which is a natural side effect of working muscles in a way they have not been worked before. Some muscle soreness is actually a really good thing, and you will learn to actually enjoy, or at least, appreciate, this type of pain. It usually is bad the next day, worse the day after that, but recovery is usually very rapid after that. A suggestion would be to work out Monday, Wednesday and Friday, giving yourself two recovery days a week before starting the cycle over again. Also, feel free to add in more activities like walking the dog or hiking, etc, if you feel up to it. You really want to work towards working out about five days a week to make significant changes in your body. Once you get to your goal weight, you can drop down to three or four days a week.

Special Tip: The Active Rest Day:

One fun way to get the weight loss happening is to make your rest days active, not passive. Call it a rest day and people automatically think about lying on the couch and watching television. But it could be so much more. An active rest day could include playing street hockey with your kids, doing a couple of hours of housework, going for a stroll in a park, going skating or hiking with a friend, playing tennis, running around the playground with your kids, taking the dog for the best walk of his life, etc. Combine fresh air, any activity and fun!

Try different, new physical activities just for a good time — move, play, laugh and dance. There are so many things you can do that are both productive in some way, and active at the same time. A great goal would be to replace one hour of television a day with ANY other kind of pastime, as long as it involves moving your body in some way. The point is to move your life away from habits that are not helpful to your goals — like watching television — to habits that help you to grow. In fact, if you got nothing out of this book except that you gave up refined sugar and stopped watching television, you would probably still be ecstatic with the results in six months from now!

Remember that the point is to get past The Discomfort Zone - the first few days and weeks when your subconscious mind is telling you to knock off all the changes already! The fear monger that keeps telling you how scary this all is. Ignore that voice — it's not trying to help you, it's just trying to keep things the same because that's what it believes is safe. In about four to six weeks, that little voice inside your head will get quieter, while all the positive benefits you are getting will be at the forefront of your mind and spirit. You can do it.

After week one, add one more workout to your routine.

After week two, check your weight and evaluate your progress. How many days a week are you working out? Remember, five days a week is best if you are trying to lose weight. Can you get in five workouts during weeks three and four? Remember that once you hit your goals, you can drop down to three to four workouts a week — a maintenance schedule.

So to recap — for 30 days do the following every single day:

* Meditate

* Have your list of goals taped to the fridge and look at them daily, along with your vision board

* Practice your visualization exercises

* Affirmations — say them often, and every day

* Stick to three meals and two snacks a day, limit refined sugar and no eating after 7 pm

* At least three of the seven days, do any kind of mild to moderate activity, class or workout, that lasts at least 20 minutes, but preferably 30 to 45 minutes. It should

make you sweat and raise your heart rate and you should feel some minor soreness the next day

* On the days in between workouts, practice active rest activities — including walks, housework, hobbies like golf, play at the playground with the kids, organize some closets in your house, chop wood, stroll around a downtown and step into the shops, walk to get some groceries and carry them home, etc.

• Cut out at least one hour of television each day, if you watch television — replace it with any other kind of activity, provided it forces you to move around, even a little.

* After two weeks re-evaluate: work towards five workouts and one active rest day a week; one pound a week weight loss is considered a healthy rate to lose at — are you there? If not, make some adjustments

* If you cheat or miss a day, do NOT give up — you have not failed if you stumble. Get up and start over the next day. Keep going, and don't give up on yourself.

* At the end of every day of the first 30 days, take a very conscious few minutes to sit quietly and go back over the day in your mind. First, point out the three best things that happened to you that day. Next, note any times that you did not succeed as you wanted to — plan out how you can do better the next day without laying any blame on yourself. Finally, practice

visualizing how you will look and feel in just a few weeks from now, when you are losing weight and feeling great! Feel how that feels and feel gratitude towards it in the moment. Tell yourself how grateful you are that you have reached your fitness goals as if you are already there — because you are! Getting started is the hardest part, and you have done that now.

Phase two of your fitness routine:

After four to six weeks on this program, change and an increase in intensity will be needed to kick up your burn and also to prevent boredom and provide muscle confusion so your body continues to work hard to adapt to the load you are putting on it. Time to incorporate weights. While earlier on I did say that lifting light weights is no way to start off a program for an overweight person, lifting weights is an excellent way to build muscle mass and give you a nice toned look. Lifting weights in not generally considered cardio, although it does burn calories and when you do compound exercises quickly with little rest in between, you can turn weight lifting into a High Intensity Interval Training routine.

If you have the money and time, go ahead and pay for a trainer to get you going with a routine. Just so you are aware, most average trainers are going to start you off with the same routine I am about to give you — so unless you really feel that you need that other person motivating you, you can simply look over this basic workout routine and google exercises to match. I recommend free weights over machines as much as possible. Before you do exercises, watch videos that show you proper form. Start with a lower weight and higher reps, then increase the weight gradually and decrease the reps. Ultimately, you want to end up doing 2 to 3 sets of 8 to 12 reps on most exercises, and the last two or three reps of every set should be difficult to do or you actually go to failure, meaning you simply cannot do another rep. This is called overload — overloading muscles causes them to tear and grow, and that's how body builders get their muscles. But you have to lift very heavy and hard to look like them. Your results will be moderate toning, unless you decide to body-build, and good for you if you do!

Squats: the general rule of thumb when you are doing a workout with weights is to start with your biggest muscle groups and work your way down. Squats are one of the most effective lower body exercises you can do, although they actually involve many other muscles that assist in stabilizing you both in the down and up phase. Squats primarily work your butt muscle (gluteus maximus) your front thigh muscles (quadriceps) and your calf muscles (soleus). There are literally dozens of different types of squats you can do, so go ahead and google or UTube squats and watch a few examples. It's good to switch up the kind of squats you do regularly to confuse your muscles into working harder and growing — change your stance, use bars sometimes, and dumb bells other times, try sumo (very wide leg) squats, change your grip, etc — but always include some type of squat in your routine.

To balance your workout, you need to work one muscle, then it's opposite — also known as the agonist and antagonist — one works while the other is passive, then vice versa. Just think always of balance — when you work the front, you need to work the back.

After squats, work the back of your thighs (hamstrings). Dead lifts, hamstring curls and ball pulls are all excellent for this muscle group. However, do not attempt dead lifts if you have neck and back pain, and if you do start performing dead lifts, start with a very light bar until your form improves, then increase the weight. Again, google these exercises for proper form first.

Next work out your chest (pectorals) by doing chest presses with either a bar or dumbbells, or dumb bell flies, or any type of push up, or cable flyes — there are other options, but again, mix it up. Change your exercises regularly to build strength and endurance. Push ups are great because they effectively work the chest, require no equipment and are a very good litmus test to see how high your fitness level is. While at first you might be doing push ups from your knees — eventually you will do regular push ups, and then several sets of regular push ups, then maybe push ups with your feet elevated on a bench. Simple exercises are sometimes the best!

We've worked our chest, so we need to work its opposite — the back. When doing back exercises in particular, we need to use proper form, increase weight gradually, pay attention to our bodies and any pain signals we receive, and perform reps slowly. A good rule of thumb when doing any weight training exercise is to stop and re-set if you feel unusual or unexpected pain during an exercise — if after re-setting and trying the same exercise twice, you feel that same pain, stop and switch to a different exercise. You don't have to be a trainer to be able to discern the difference between discomfort because you are working hard and pain that is coming from an injury, overuse, improper form or another issue. Don't ignore this type of pain.

Back exercises that are especially good include pulling moves such as lat pull downs and seated rows. Bent over rows and bent over flyes are also good. If you are working out at home, you would only need a couple of dumbbells to effectively work your back.

Once you get comfortable with weight lifting, you can add many more exercises that include shoulder moves, biceps, triceps, calves , etc. But to start with, just work on your primal movements: leg muscles front and back, push and pull moves, and abdominals.

Abdominals - do me a favour — give up crunches permanently. They are the least effective abdominal exercise and in that sense, a time waster. Google dead bug, V ball pass, planks, and/or use an ab wheel. The point is your abdominals should be sore the next day after a good series of sets of the above mentioned exercises.

I remember a trainer I knew said to me once that — everyone actually has six-pack abs: it's just that most people have a layer of fat overtop — the more of the fat that you remove, the more of your six-pack is revealed! It's the same with you entire body — so you do have a beautiful toned body, it's just underneath a layer of insulation that you can remove if you follow this program and stick to it for life.

If you commit to your eating plan and a variation of the above program for two solid months, I guarantee you will see changes to your body, your energy level and your self esteem. Soon, you will crave the rush of physical exercise, and the growing number of compliments you will receive.

It's also crucial to find a time of the day to fit in exercise that works for you and fits into your lifestyle. A young woman I work with who has a toddler brings her running gear to work and takes her hour lunch as a long run - BRAVO - she knows that once she gets home, there is very little me time, and she has structured her life accordingly. She is a smart lady and she looks great. Find these kinds of solutions and work with a flow that makes your life easier and not harder. Most people know whether they are morning people or not. Personally, my favourite time to go out for a run and hit the gym is around 7:30 am - I have no idea why this works for me, it just does. I have a friend who hits the gym before work at 5:00 am at least three days a week. I personally think she's nuts, but … it works for her and fits into her lifestyle. Don't try to force anything that doesn't feel right for you. Go with your natural energy levels — that way you are more likely to stick with your routine long-term.

My friend who does the 5 am workouts loves her routine and also looks fantastic! She has the satisfaction of starting work at 8 am having already done her workout, showered and basically gotten the hard part of her day over with. No matter how sideways her work day goes, no one can take that from her. She goes to be early and wakes up early. This is what works for her as a busy single mom with a full-time job and other commitments. So you see it doesn't matter when you work out, just that you find a time that doesn't make you want to puke, and that you can do regularly each week without screwing up the rest of your life.

Chapter 14

Fire up your body: muscle confusion and changing routines

Whether you are just starting a new workout program, or plateauing just a few pounds from your goal, or just feeling bored and tired of your gym and cardio routine — the solution is the same — you need to change exercises, order, weight and activities regularly — every four to six weeks — to continue achieving results.

Our muscles are as clever as our minds, and they adapt to any load placed upon them over time. That is why a painter can climb ladders and roll walls around all day, every day, and not feel like all of his muscles are like lead. If I went to work as a painter and matched that worker stroke for stroke for 12 hours straight, I probably wouldn't be able to move for two or three days.

In other words, our bodies get used to the demands we make on them, provided we are working the same muscles on a regular basis. That is why we get sore the day after a new workout or after we have just started working out for the first time or after a long break. The pain normally gets a little worse on the second day, then dissipates quickly after that. However, if you stick with your same routine, you will find the soreness gets less and less, until, like a lot of well trained and fit people, they just don't get sore anymore. While it's great not to feel that kind of pain in one way, that is actually a sign that your body has completely adapted to the activity you are doing, and you will likely slow down on your progress towards: losing weight, gaining muscle, or whatever goals you might be working towards.

And so, it is necessary to change your routine regularly — for example — switch from straight running to fartleking or intervals (running slow, then fast, for set periods of time). Switch from walking to hiking trails for a few weeks. Switch up at least half of your weight training exercises — for example — switch from standing dumbbell curls to concentration curls; from tricep kick-backs to dips on a bench; from barbell squats to sumo squats; you get the picture — there are many variations of exercises that train the muscles of the body — although you may think changing HOW you do the exercise isn't going to change the result — the soreness you will feel the next day will turn you into a believer.

Experts are still not sure what causes Delayed Onset of Muscle Soreness, but we do know it is predictable. You will get sore when by push your body beyond the limits it is used to. This is also the reason why some people continue to start and stop working out, get frustrated, and eventually give up all together. They get on track for a couple of weeks, get into excuse mode, then stop for a week or two, and end up right back where they started again, feeling really sore without seeing results. Really, they are dooming themselves to continually starting all over again almost every month or two — until they either give up entirely, or finally realize that you really need to make a full commitment to getting into shape and truly putting in at least three to six months into it — enough time to see some measurable results. This is also enough time to begin to see some of those longer term health benefits — wider Range of Motion and flexibility, improved heart health and cardiovascular fitness, more energy and happiness and a more positive attitude towards the future.

This process of changing things up is called muscle confusion — it literally means that you are changing things up in a way your body wasn't expecting, and it is the key to making continued progress once you get into the swing of working out. And though it may seem strange to you at first, I can almost guarantee that you will learn to strangely enjoy feeling sore muscles that come the day after a really good workout — it makes you feel sure that you have torn muscles fibres which you know will make them — and you — stronger and better. It is by changing things up, by increasing weight, by never doing the same thing over and over for a long period of time, that you will continue to make gains in whatever direction you wish to make them.

Muscle memory is another important thing to know about your amazing body. If you were fit for a period of time in the past and then slipped into a state non-activity for a period of time, it will actually be easier for you to get back into that same shape again than it would be for someone who has literally never exercised regularly (all other factors being equal). Your muscles actually do carry the memory of the load you used to be able to place on them and will quickly adapt again to assist you in getting back in that shape again. Isn't it fantastic to know that our muscles are saving this information for us? The body is truly an amazing machine!

Some other facts to keep in mind — muscles do not turn into fat if you stop working out. However, you may gain weight because your calorie intake will outweigh your calorie burning output and you will likely begin to store more fat on your body around your muscles. But the muscles themselves are the same as they were when you were in shape, except weaker and smaller. Remember again that to burn off fat that accumulates over the muscles is mainly done by performing cardiovascular exercise — in a slow to moderate pace on a regular basis, which creates the fire that burns fat.

Lifting weights is crucial to strengthen and tone muscles and also burns calories, although it is not considered "cardio". However, you can sequence your exercises into compound movements done quickly with little rest between sets, and you will burn fat during a weight training session.

One piece of VERY important advice I would like to give everyone who plans to start weight training for fitness and fun, is to learn the basics of how all the exercises are performed properly and how to correctly use all the machines in the gym **BEFORE** you ever start a routine. And by that I do not mean have a friend show you — because they may only pass on their bad habits and bad form to you, which won't help you in the least.

Watch some UTube videos by reputable trainers, or hire a trainer or ask a qualified gym employee or manager to take you through all the machines once (it will take about an hour) and free weights in the gym or ask an employee at your new gym to show you how the equipment works. I can't stress this enough. The reasons why are plentiful but let me name a few: firstly, if you start using equipment wrong or performing reps incorrectly you could quickly injure yourself, and then you will be forced to stop working out, possibly for a long time. Neck and back injuries can become chronic, so you don't want to cause yourself this kind of harm. Proper form prevents many injuries that take place at the gym.

Secondly, once you start using bad form during an exercise, it becomes very difficult to change to the correct form, because the wrong way has become engrained in you. In fact, I have seen trainers approach gym members who are clearly doing an exercise completely wrong and after being told so by a professional, they just keep doing it the wrong way because that's what they are used to and are comfortable with.

Thirdly, Using poor form, such as swinging the weights instead of controlling them or simply dropping them on the negative part of the rep instead of lowering them in a controlled fashion, will practically negate any benefit you would get from the exercise, and you might as well be sitting at home on the couch. Your movements on the down and up phases of any movement should be slow and controlled at every stage, and you should never use momentum or fling weights around in any way, shape or form.

Jeez, doesn't this whole chapter seem like just plain old common sense? But you would be amazed to see how many people, women in particular — are afraid to add weight training to their routine because they have no idea what the benefits are, and how fun weight training can be. And you would be even more amazed to see learn how many people are working out in gyms and simply not performing the exercises properly, not lifting nearly as much weight as they could or should be, and not using controlled movements. It is not a wonder that so many people get frustrated and give up the gym — they either don't see results and don't know why, get injured and don't want to return, or feel embarassed because they don't know how to use the equipment properly and so they just don't come back.

So to re-cap:

1. Change things up every month or two to confuse your muscles to help them grow

2. Remember that feeling somewhat sore for one to two days after a challenging workout is actually a good thing

3. You muscles remember their best shape and want to bring you back to it

4. Learn proper form before performing any exercise, do not fling weights or use momentum, and control your movements on the way up and down — never drop them — focus on controlling all phases of the movement

Chapter 15

Exercise Reverses the Aging Process

If you need an even better motivation to begin and stick with a workout program, how about this: exercise is scientifically proven to help reverse the aging process, particularly the changes our bodies go through after the age of 30. Isn't that an incentive to get out there and move? The point of this book is to assist you in believing in yourself and using the power of your mind to control the actions of your body. And another great thing that helps us is to imprint positive messages into our subconscious to propel us forward. One of the messages you need to be telling yourself during meditation and visualization is that: I am staying young because I exercise. And the really amazing thing is: It's true!

Human Growth Hormone (HGH) is a key component that is responsible for our rapid growth during childhood years. Think for a moment about growth spurts that happened with you or your children, which is a perfect example of how HGH works in the human body. This magic bullet assists us in the repair of tissue and is present in high amounts until we reach later adulthood.

The fact of the matter is that, when we hit about 30 years of age, our levels of HGH plummet to as low as 20 per cent of their highest levels during childhood and early adulthood. After this time, our bodies can no longer rely on high levels of this amazing hormone to help with tissue regeneration, and as a result, we begin to not only age, but to age far more rapidly than we would if our levels of HGH stayed the same, or at least didn't drop so dramatically. It really is akin to the Fountain of Youth.

Did you know that studies have proven that exercise, in particular High Intensity Interval Training - actually helps your body naturally produce higher levels of HGH, which in turn assists in reversing some of the more negative physical affects of aging/inactivity: namely reversing the speed at which our muscles weaken and atrophy. Isn't this incredible information to have? Just think, many of you are aging far more quickly than you should or could be, and for no reason other than you are not keeping your bodies moving.

Try not to think of this bodily process as scary, think of it as enlightening and an opportunity for change. This book is about getting positive messages into your conscious and subconscious mind about the power of fitness, which will in turn help motivate you. I want you to install a barrage of positive feelings about yourself and about exercise into your filing cabinet, to replace any negative thoughts about yourself or about exercise that you may have.

* Exercise will make me young again.

* Exercise is fun and good for me.

* I love the way my body feels when it is being active.

* I am in control of my body, and that is how it will be for life.

Back to creating more of that youth hormone inside your body — So once you have begun whatever exercise program that you feel good doing and have been at it a few weeks and are feeling like a challenge, try incorporating some HIIT, provided you do not have a medical condition that contradicts periods of intense activity within your workouts.

The fantastic thing about this kind of training is that you only need to do it about three times a week for 20 minutes per session to get the full benefits of boosting your HGH and, in essence, fighting back against the natural aging process. Not that any of us can win, but the longer we can feel strong, the better our quality of life will be, and the happier we can expect to be. In fact, it is not recommended that you perform high intensity exercise more often than three times a week, so mix it up with some longer, low to medium intensity cardio sessions and/or classes, and/or weight training sessions at the gym, or even just brisk walks for 45 minutes or longer on the in-between days. Whatever makes you feel good and pushes you ahead towards your goals! I take at least one full day off from either the gym or running every week — to give my body a full 24 hours without being strained in any way.

Here's how to plan your own high intensity workout for HGH building.

1. Warm up: this is crucial — three to five minutes of marching on the spot, knee lifts, light jumping jacks, arm rotations, etc — warming up serves many functions, it

gets synovial fluid moving in your joints which lubricates and prepares them to work; increases heart rate in preparation for exercise; warms up the body, allowing for free Range of Motion with the risk of injury; and mentally prepares you for the workout.

Create a circuit for yourself with anywhere from five to 10 stations — or just create a list of exercises you can do on the spot using just your body weight — the beauty of this routine is you actually don't need any equipment at all! There are dozens of moves you can choose from but here's a list of possible exercises:

Bicycle crunches

Box jumps

Burpees

Jumping jacks

Push ups

Sumo squats

Side lunges

Running on the spot

Lateral jumps

Squat jumps

High knees

Mountain climbers

Medicine ball throws

Planks

Push ups with rotation

Jab/cross/jab (or any punching combination done fast)

Eccentric push ups

Plank jacks

During each exercise, go as hard and fast as you can for 30 to 45 seconds, rest for 60 to 90 seconds, then go on to the next station or exercise, and continue on with this pattern until you have hit the 20 minute mark. Do not forget to spend five to ten minutes cooling down after a HIIT, it's vital to slowly get your heart rate back to normal, instead of abruptly stopping.

Tips:

Stairs present a great tool for high intensity workouts either indoors or outdoors. You can simply do stair intervals, or layer stairs with other exercises in your home made circuit.

When laying out your exercises for the routine try to incorporate moves for as many different muscle groups as possible — think upper body and lower body, side to side movements and forwards and back movements; Jumping movements and pushing and pulling movements. Add one abdominal move but not more than one, or you might be too sore the next day.

Chapter 16
Conquering life's Mental Traps

There's a funny little tradition at my office that I consider an amazing bi-weekly experiment on the human condition around "sinful" or "bad" foods. Every second Friday (Payday Friday), one of our employees faithfully brings in an entire box of donuts of many different flavours to the office and places them on a table just a few feet in front of my desk. I have honestly never had one of his donuts (or half or even a bite of one), but I have watched, week after week, as (mainly) the woman who work on my floor (oh, and couple that come up from downstairs) practically throw themselves on the ground in a perverse inner battle, trying to decide whether or not they are going to eat one donut.

"Oh my god, donuts!"

"Oh, Julia, should I have one or not?"

"No! Keep them away from me!"

"I'm going to get a knife" (to cut and eat half the donut … only to come back an hour later and guiltily take the other half back to their office to finish it off).

"I'm not going to have one, I just want to look at them!"

"I'm so weak!"

I find it hilarious and totally fascinating. The agony and ecstasy of what I call "Unscheduled Food." Unscheduled food is food brought into the office, or to a party, to into your home, by a person who is trying to do something nice and has good intentions. Food: treats and sweets especially — are one of the easiest things to buy for co-workers, or for a party or gathering, that you know they will like, aside from coffee or wine. Plus, the sugar gives people a short-term rush of energy and happiness (for about 15 minutes, that is, until they crash again).

The problem is that unscheduled food appears often in a lot of situations: at weekly meetings, all holidays, people's birthdays, summer BBQs - you get the picture — when you add it all up it's at least a weekly and sometimes a daily event. Take for a powerful example the weeks leading up to Christmas.

Honestly, if you want to make fitness a priority and you want to lose weight, you really need to make a firm decision to never or rarely eat unscheduled food, sorry it's a bummer. Or if you must occasionally indulge, plan out when you are going to take part in eating unscheduled food at the office or a party, and try to make that a habit you only every once in a blue moon. I myself always take part in our office's annual Christmas pot luck. There's turkey and potatoes and all sorts of desserts, and I eat whatever I want. That's literally the only time I eat out of routine at the office. It may seem silly and you may feel like you are depriving yourself or feeling left out at first, but if you really look around at the people who are always digging into the free food at work, you can bet that the majority of them are not in great physical condition, and are not paying conscious attention to what they put inside their bodies.

The holidays are actually kind of a funny thing: if you believe the hype created by television shows, films, commercials and advertisements seen everywhere and anywhere after Nov. 11 (and sometimes before), then you might think everyone is supposed to be carefree, happy with their families, able to afford any and all gifts and decorations …. and live in a beautifully decorated big house and … but what nonsense! The holidays are really a difficult time for most people, and it's a time when many women feel weak because they are under a tremendous amount of stress to try to make their homes the happy Christmas place that it's supposed to be. But stress equals bad eating equals missed workouts equals feeling bad, not good, about yourself.

The truth of the matter is that many people find the holidays a difficult and even a depressing time — including people who are alone, those who can't afford to keep up with their neighbours, those who don't even have homes to decorate, and people trying really hard to get fit and lose weight. After December 1 in particular, offices are littered with chocolates, cookies, tarts, pastries, cheese and cracker spreads and on and on. The problem with the holiday season is that it turns on our "unconscious eating" button and turns off our attentive habits that we may have been working on for weeks and even months! We say to ourselves, "What's the big deal? It's just a few treats and a few big meals right?" But, it is a big deal. It's a big deal because a person can gain anywhere from one to 10 pounds over just a few weeks, depending on how much they eat and drink, and to what extent they give up on exercise over the holiday season. I'm not trying to be a party pooper, but really, are the holidays about how much you can eat and drink? No, they are not. They are traditionally a time to gather with family, to show kindness and gratitude towards each other and to spend a little downtime in the comfort of our own homes.

A lovely lady I once worked with felt she had to buy a new gaming station for her son, even though he had one already. But this one was newer and better — however it cost her almost $400 and that didn't include any of the games! It's not a wonder that overeating is rampant over the holiday season — it's really a symptom of the extreme emotional and financial stress people place themselves under.

So how can you stop yourself from going over the top over Christmas and other holiday times? Here's a few simple tips that I hope you will take to heart starting next November:

If you can make no other change, at least stop eating unconsciously — that means don't pick up food as you walk by the lunch room and eat it before you've even thought about it or whether you even really want it. Also, try not to snack while watching television or movies, when you really aren't paying attention to what or how much you are putting in your mouth. Don't eat in the car while driving, because you won't even taste your food or have the chance to enjoy it. Basically, stop eating unless you are sitting down to eat and do nothing else, and you are being clear and honest with yourself about what it is you are putting inside you. And by the way, these tips work all year long, not just during the holidays.

Secondly, do NOT give up on your workout routine — just don't! Yes, there will be times you cannot work out due to social commitments and/or the gym being closed or possibly weather conditions. But really make an effort to continue working out normally on all the days you can leading up until the week of Christmas or whatever holiday. Understand that by not working out and eating unconsciously you can do a lot of damage to your progress — not to mention your self esteem. After a couple of weeks of not working out, you lose gains quickly, and you will suffer for that when you try to get back on track. I remember my holiday to Antigua two years ago with my husband. I had high hopes of going for runs and doing body weight workouts, I had even planned out a few routines. But instead, I decided to drink on the beach every single day and lay out on the beach every day! After we got home, I went back to the gym the next morning and tried to do my regular run and weight routine. Not only could I only do about 75 per cent of what I normally did every day, but I was **KILLER** sore for three or four days after and really suffered. If I had done just three or four workouts during those two weeks, I would have saved myself a lot of suffering.

Starting over is never easy, so try to keep up your momentum as much as possible.

If, as many people are, you are invited to more than one dinner over the holidays — decide which one will be your "gorge" and only overeat at that one function. It sounds silly but nowadays due to blended families, divorces and extended families, about 75 per cent of people are invited to or attend at least two full-blown turkey dinners at every major holiday. It really does help to give yourself boundaries to live by, as opposed to just tossing everything over your shoulder. The other risk you take is really going off track, getting discouraged and giving up on yourself all together. I want you to succeed and success is for life!

In the end, it's always a good idea to stop and ask ourselves: Why am I doing this? Is this behaviour helping me become the person I want to be, or could it be hurting me instead? Taking control of your life is something no one can take away from you.

Chapter 17

Choosing a Better Reward System

Let's explore a few other facts about food. After all: what you eat is at least 50% responsible for your weight and physical fitness. Most of us can't achieve our health and fitness goals without pairing good food habits with good exercise habits.

First and foremost, human beings are mammals with some traits and tendencies that come from very deep inside our evolutionary code. We hunted and gathered, and when we had food, we ate it. Early man did not save half a woolly mammoth sandwich for later — he ate the food he could get his hands on right away and got as full as he could because he instinctually did not know when he would be able to eat again. The hunt and gather existence was so close to the edge for early man, that any thought of saving for later was non-existent.

Let's look at the example of another mammal — the domesticated dog. I am not saying that we are like dogs, obviously we are far more intelligent, capable and sophisticated. But it is interesting to note that the main way dogs are trained to do tricks is by offering a food reward. Generally, these dogs are well-fed, they don't NEED that little morsel you are giving them to sit and shake a paw, but man do they want it!

The fact is that we as human beings have also developed the use food as a reward when "training" children to behave, both at home and out in public. Most of us have had experiences such as being in the grocery store as a young child and grabbing for or asking for a candy bar. Mom responds with, "Ok little Julia, you can have that chocolate bar but only if you are a good girl and behave and walk with mommy while we are doing the grocery shopping." Similarly at home, if there is a dessert to follow dinner, many parents tell their children, "Look, there's a piece of cake for you for your dessert, but only if you finish everything on your plate."

Halloween is basically a celebration that has morphed into children dressing up and walking around in the dark and cold and knocking on strangers doors: all to get candy and lots of it!Are you getting the impression now that food represents a very potent and powerful reward for us that has been set up since childhood? There's no denying it. This is why many new fad diets offer up cheat meals or even cheat days, to help attract new dieters by promising them if they can just be good for six days, they can eat whatever they want on day seven. It's like Halloween once a week!

While there is nothing wrong with trying this approach if it really works for you, I would suggest that a better strategy would be to work at not using food as a reward nearly as much, and to make a conscious effort to choose other types of rewards and to really feel the different kind of pleasure they can give you. After all, eating food provides only a short-term rush of pleasure, and if it is too much food, it can produce a much longer period of pain than the pleasure you got from it in the first place. As the Buddha aptly put it, no matter what food looks like when you put it into your mouth, it all comes out looking the same way — and it's not very beautiful. In other words, try not putting so much importance on the pleasures of eating, which are fleeting.

There are other types of rewards that you can offer yourself instead of a cheat day. By the way, during an entire day of unabated eating you can actually consume enough calories to set you back an entire week. A person who binges for an entire day can eat 10,000 or more calories, which if not burned off equals almost three pounds worth. Have you ever considered that cheat days actually keep you on a perpetual cycle of lose and gain, gain and lose? Have you also considered that the purveyors of these diets WANT you to stay on that roller coaster so that you can remain on their program? Ask yourself how, over the long term, does this really serve you? And as a final thought, this type of conditioning builds up a strong desire in you to regularly binge, even if you never were a binge-eater before. This is really not a habit you want to develop for life.

Examples of other types of rewards you can give yourself for training hard and for reaching your short and long-term goals:

* A new piece of workout gear (shoes, sports bra, tights, YAH!)

* A stop at the local pool for a good long soak in the whirlpool looking great in your bathing suit

* A simple glass of really good white wine with a friend at a nice lounge in the afternoon — a low cal indulgence.

* Spending time trying on old clothes to see which ones fit you again — that's not only fun but really inspiring as well.

* Calling up a good friend and telling her about your success and hearing the praise — you need this!

* Planning a future getaway around your fitness goals, such as a week in Mexico - isn't that better than one day of pigging out a week?

* A massage and pedicure at a local resort or spa

* Meet someone for coffee that hasn't seen you in a few weeks, and soak in the compliments!

Take a really relaxing yoga stretch class or meditation class to really wind down and get your thoughts on what is important

Buy three or four current fitness magazines and comb them for inspirational stories and all kinds of tips on exercise and clean eating — honestly, it's fun and helps energize you

Chapter 18

Master the Subconscious;
the Body will Follow

By the time you have gotten through the first 30 days of your program, you should feel momentum kicking in. You're on the bike, you've pedalled and wobbled a bit, you speed up on the peddles and now you are coasting down the flat road with no one on it! The best advice I or anyone else could give you is to just keep going. Don't ever give into excuses and do not stop visualizing your success and meditating. These are excellent tools that you will use for the rest of your life.

Remember that the main goal here is to feel good about yourself. It's not to reach a certain weight, but to reach a certain lifestyle that works for you and makes you feel good about yourself. A lot of people get caught up in the gain weight, lose weight, gain weight cycle, and it makes them feel utterly miserable and defeated a lot of the time. The trick is that once your mind is strong and on board for change, you are guaranteed to stick with your program. And don't forget about the power momentum has — once you get your second wind, things will start to happen quickly and it will almost feel as if they are happening all on their own. Your results will get more dramatic, yet the process will feel easier and more fun. Once you reach this stage you will know it. It's pretty easy to stay in a state of momentum for long periods of time, and it feels really good to be there.

One of the best things you can do after you have used this program to get yourself back on track is to help other people in your life do the same. Share this information freely with family members, friends, co-workers and anyone else you may feel will benefit from it. Helping other people is why we are here on this planet. It is the reason I wrote this book and the reason we were created. It's easy to get caught up in our own problems and our own little inner worlds. But what you will find is that once you start helping others, it enriches your life and makes you feel happier, which in turn brings you more momentum to keep you feeling better about your own life as well.

In closing, I send you my blessings and welcome your feedback. I truly hope this book starts you on a journey that ends in you looking, feeling and being, a happy and fit human being.

This is Trainer Julia signing off: Have a Fit Day!